Ultrasound Causation

~ *for* ~

Microcephaly and Zika virus

The Hypothesis

Part A

by

Jim West

ISBN 978-1-941719-08-4
Library of Congress Control Number: 2017944068

Publisher's Cataloging-in-Publication Data

West, Jim, 1947-
Ultrasound Causation for Microcephaly and Zika virus:
The Hypothesis (Part A)
pages cm
Includes bibliographical references.
ISBN: 978-1-941719-08-4 (paperback b/w)
1. Ultrasonics in obstetrics. 2. Ultrasonic imaging.
3. Medicine—Research. I. Title.
RG527.5.U48 W47 2017
618.207543—dc23 2017944068

Disclaimer

Those seeking medical advice should consult medical professionals without delay. Verify this work with professionals. I am not an authority or an official expert.

This work encourages reasonable discussion of the contradictions throughout the history of medical and therapeutic ultrasound. Presently there appears to be is no sufficient authoritative public forum for resolution of these contradictions.

This is based on scientific authority. Nevertheless, any views derived from this work are technically inconclusive pending trusted authoritative review at a high level. There is an implicit subjunctive throughout any of my work, where everything is subject to higher confirmation.

Though the foundation is strong, nothing is written in stone. Corrections or suggestions are welcome at harvoa.org/contact

Intent can never be known but if stated or implied, that would have been as a mere working position for this hypothetical review.

The application of my work to any specific human case must remain moot due to the complexities and randomness of diagnostic ultrasound (DUS) exposure and biological responses.

Acknowledgement

The Townsend Letter, Anthony Brink, Maria Schiaffino, Mitchel Cohen and NoSpray Coalition, *Nexus Magazine*, *GreenMedInfo*, Gary Krasner, John Wantling, The Perth Group, Chris Rawlins, June Segal, Eugene Semons (deceased), Jesús García Blanca of *Discovery Salud*, Amy Worthington, John Scudamore, Adam Crabb, *Global Freedom Network*. Special thanks to Ingri Cassell of Vaccine Liberation.

Thanks to Jon Rappoport for his immediate and strong criticism of the Brazil microcephaly epidemic, and to Claus Jensen for his research and comraderie.

Dedication

This book is sincerely dedicated to those at *The Telemedicine Network* in NE Brazil, the eye of the storm.

Zika virus is guilty until proven innocent.

Dr. Anthony Costello, Director of
Maternal, Newborn, Child and Adolescent Health at
The World Health Organization (2/2/2016)

Contents

Preface

Because this is literary criticism, quote marks contain only the original text, i.e., punctuation such as periods and commas are placed in quotes only when they are in the original.

See the Glossary. In addition to pertinent science jargon, a few terms have been modified for this topic.

[Brackets] are my annotations. **Bold** and *italicized* text is my emphasis. Graphs and images are mine, rendered from topical data, unless otherwise noted.

Join the email list at harvoa.org for notifications of new material, corrections, and updates: harvoa.org/contact/

Introduction

Empirical base

DUS is the acronym for "Diagnostic ultrasound", commonly known as a prenatal examination procedure.

THIS IS DUS BOOK 2

This book presents an incredible *Hypothesis* — that DUS is the cause of the recent microcephaly epidemic in NE Brazil, an epidemic falsely blamed on "Zika virus".

This book presents some of the many inevitable pragmatic discussions that must follow the implications of DUS Book 1. The tone of this book is direct and unapologetic because it rests on empirical evidence.

This volume's short name is "Part A" (of three Parts). It critically reviews terminology. It critically reviews the epidemic and reveals the actual character.

EMPIRICAL BASE: DUS BOOK 1

The prior book, DUS Book 1, is the foundation, published in May 2015, titled, *50 Human Studies, A New Bibliography.* That book has been generally confirmed with positive comments, the lack of any negative comments, and consistent public and professional interest. It can meet any scientific challenge.

The prior book carefully reviews ultrasound studies that have been ignored, overlooked, or dismissed, i.e., the Western animal studies exemplified by Cachon (1981), Liebeskind (1979-1982), Anderson and Barrett (1979-1981), Ang (2006), Ellisman (1987), Saad and Williams (1982), and it presents an unprecedented discovery of Chinese Human Studies (CHS), and thus its title, *A New Bibliography*.

Many supportively engaged in discussion, including scientists and medical professionals. Medicos (mainstream medical practitioners, including most midwives), mainstream journalists and wire services are generally quiet. Independent journals have published strong articles. There are no negative responses to date.

The CHS are modern human fetal studies, conducted at exposures often much lower than clinical. They found DUS damage to cellular ultrastructures, DNA, chromatins (DNA packaging), cell nuclei, membranes and mitochondria. Also found damaged were ovaries, ova, embryos, neurons, testicles, sperm, chorionic villi, immune system, kidney, pituitary, thyroid and cornea. Earlier cell studies found damage heritable through generations.

Praise for DUS Book 1

Jon Rappoport, Investigative Journalist

> *...Jim West... his meticulous analysis has turned the establishment on its head. If I were the king of Pulitzers, I would give him a dozen. He is what truly deep reporting is all about.*

Eitan Kimmel, PhD, Dept of Biomedical Engineering, Technion Institute, one of the world's premier research centers.

> *Your book is wonderful. You found the human studies. Chapter five is terrifying! I wish I were wrong.*

Sam Milham, MD, MPH, former epidemiologist for New York State, professor, author, and EMF scientist.

> *Great job. Your book is doing a valuable service to the childbearing public... You just cannot expose a fetus to this much energy without doing harm. For example, see Newnham (1993).*

Zvonko Hočevar, LLT Dr, Ljubljana University Medical Centre

> *Congratulations for your book and your courage in presenting this topic to public. Heartfelt thanks! I did my Doctorate of Science, finding 'no evidence based medicine' supporting 'safety' of ultrasound in IVF (in vitro fertilization) procedures.*

Manuel F. Casanova, MD, Vice Chair for Research in the Department of Psychiatry and Behavioral Sciences at University of Louisville.

> *This is important work. Attention must be brought upon the subject. Ultrasound is more than taking pretty pictures of babies. We are learning about side effects and mechanisms of potential harms that have not been the object of safety studies, least regulations. You have brought together the field by summarizing many different areas that bear on the subject, from physics to biology and medicine. Your writing should raise awareness in the layperson, that ultrasound is a "buyers beware" market. That before the glacial pace of our government moves to take action it is*

their responsibility to become informed and take adequate decisions.

Dr. Casanova is a prominent neuroscientist, with groundbreaking research in the field of cortical neurocircuitry, e.g., brain minicolumns. See "The Neuropathology of Autism" in *Brain Pathology*[1] and other work.[2,3,4]

William O'Brien, Jr, PhD, prominent ultrasound scientist, author, former President of AIUM (American Institute of Ultrasound in Medicine), former Chair of AIUM Bioeffects Committee, and Director of Bioacoustics Research Laboratory.

O'Brien authored a commentary of JZhang (2002) in response to my lobbying. Extract:

The study, JZhang (2002) was relatively well done and documented with a dose-effect response... The study needs to be reproduced... 13 mW/cm2 is really low... The finding is important... the SPTA [intensity] levels do not

---

[1] Manuel F. Casanova, "The Neuropathology of Autism," *Brain Pathology* 17, no. 4 (October 1, 2007): 422–33, doi:10.1111/j.1750-3639.2007.00100.x.

[2] E. L. Williams and M. F. Casanova, "Potential Teratogenic Effects of Ultrasound on Corticogenesis: Implications for Autism," *Medical Hypotheses* 75, no. 1 (July 2010): 53–58, doi:10.1016/j.mehy.2010.01.027.

[3] Emily L. Williams and Manuel F. Casanova, "Reassessment of Teratogenic Risk from Antenatal Ultrasound," *Translational Neuroscience* 4, no. 1 (March 1, 2013): 81–87.

[4] Emily L. Williams and Manuel F. Casanova, "Ultrasound and Autism: How Disrupted Redox Homeostasis and Transient Membrane Porosity Confer Risk," in *Studies on Psychiatric Disorders*, ed. Anna Dietrich-Muszalska, Ved Chauhan, and Sylvain Grignon, Oxidative Stress in Applied Basic Research and Clinical Practice (Springer New York, 2015), 373–92, doi:10.1007/978-1-4939-0440-2_18.

support [the thermal] view [i.e., a non-thermal mechanism is supported].

Stephanie Seneff, PhD, Senior Research Scientist, MIT

I read your book and I was fascinated by it! ...ultrasound as a possible danger during pregnancy... I am now much more aware.

Tedd Koren, DC, noted chiropractor

Thanks so much. I can always depend on you for great info. You are a true seeker of truth.

Kelly Brogan, MD, author, speaker

Human studies condemn ultrasound! Jim West has compiled the largest bibliography of human ultrasound studies.

Gary Krasner, Coalition for Informed Choice

Jim West is the leading independent researcher of disease causation from chemical exposure. Now he has written a ground-breaking book that documents the inconvenient facts about the dangers of ultrasound. Parents and medical professionals should reconsider the cost/benefit of ultrasound.

Ramiel Nagel, author of *Healing Our Children*

There is clear evidence that ultrasounds during pregnancy can change fetal tissues. Jim West dug up this impossible to find evidence to make it obviously clear that we should not be haphazardly using video ultrasounds when less invasive technologies can be used.

Amy Worthington, wi-cancer.info

> *I have read this book slowly and every page is marked and underlined and highlighted. It is brilliant the way it ties together so many loose strings and exposes the lies. In my opinion, this book is THE most important work of our times.*

Nexus Magazine

> *Western scientific and medical professionals do not seem to be aware of the many human studies that have been conducted in China which clearly indicate damage from the use of diagnostic ultrasound. It is time that they examined this new compilation of research.*

Russell B. Olinsky, M.S. Environmental Specialist

> *Jim West should get a Goethe Prize.... The ramifications should be huge, but alas I do not' expect change due to vested interests.*

Daniel Maciejewski

> *This is a well written book on a crucially important subject... Even before reading this book, I was convinced that prenatal ultrasound is leading to the boom in autism and other developmental disorders in children. After reading this book, any doubt I had about the damaging effects of ultrasound are gone. Jim West does a wonderful job of not only presenting the research, but providing a framework for understanding what is going on.*

Michael Ellner, HEAL-NY

Jim West's passion and skill for finding, checking, exposing bogus medical facts and the economic, political, and social forces that drive and protect conventional medical practice is legendary among alternative health care activists.

—Overview—

1 | Medical Words

Orwellianism

This chapter introduces medical words relevant to the microcephaly epidemic.

Medical words can only be understood through a skeptical process. Medicine purports to be about personal health and science, however, its language evolves through industrial interest in profit from the sales of services, pharmaceuticals, gadgets, liability protection, and an extended web of conflicted opportunities and obligations.

While many medical definitions are useful and real, others are carefully honed to make mere discussion of environmental causation impossible.

Funding research for environmental causation, especially DUS (Diagnostic Ultrasound), is marginalized, for example, consider the IACC:

> *The Interagency Autism Coordinating Committee (IACC) is a Federal advisory committee that coordinates all efforts*

within the Department of Health and Human Services (HHS) concerning autism spectrum disorder (ASD).[5]

This federal agency directs U.S. tax dollars to autism research[6] where funds go almost entirely towards the genetic causation industry, some germ causation research and little environmental research. Ultrasound is virtually unmentioned.[7]

Another example is Gardener (2011), a review of autism causation,

...a comprehensive meta-analysis... [of] the association between perinatal and neonatal factors and autism.

Gardener studied 60 factors, and like all mainstream literature, ends inconclusively. It implies risk and causation by pointing one symptom at another. Without comment, it omits medical radiation![8]

An earlier study by the same team, Gardener (2009), a meta-analysis of prenatal factors, also ends inconclusively. It exculpates X-rays and entirely omits the word "ultrasound". It does find maternal bleeding to be a factor, which happens to be a complaint from women following DUS sessions.

---

[5] "IACC | Interagency Autism Coordinating Committee," accessed March 18, 2017, https://iacc.hhs.gov/.

[6] The Interagency Autism Coordinating Committee (IACC) was originally established under the Children's Health Act of 2000 (Public Law 106-310).

[7] IACC, "2010 IACC Autism Spectrum Disorder Research Portfolio Analysis Report," 2010, http://iacc.hhs.gov/portfolio-analysis/2010/index.shtml#q3.

[8] Hannah Gardener, Donna Spiegelman, and Stephen L. Buka, "Perinatal and Neonatal Risk Factors for Autism: A Comprehensive Meta-Analysis," *Pediatrics* 128, no. 2 (August 2011): 344–55, doi:10.1542/peds.2010-1036.

Psychiatrists and psychologists often serve as point-of-sale reps for medical concepts, products and services. Their official manual for mental disorders (DSM-IV) describes basic terms.

Diagnostic and Statistical Manual of Mental Disorders (DSM IV)

The DSM defines Autism, ASD, and ADHD as mental disorders and syndromes.

DSM IV definitions

Fundamental terms applicable to any discussion of any disease are paraphrased from DSM-IV:

Symptom: An abnormal state or disease, from the Greek, meaning misfortune. Cause is not implicated.

Disorder: A cluster of symptoms, like a syndrome. Cause is not implicated.

Disease: A disorder where cause is known. This is the highest order of understanding.

Syndrome: A set of symptoms, disorders and/or conditions. Cause is not implicated.

Spectrum: A set of disorders.

Environment

Modern Medicine includes “germ” within the term “environmental”, as if germs were an environmental stressor. This is an untenable confusion. “Germs vs Environment” is an effective diagnostic dichotomy that should not be diluted.

Germ theories trigger toxic medical programs (vaccine and pesticide) without democratic process. They force by law and propaganda, toxic treatments that compound the damage of what may likely be environmental diseases.

MediLexicon defines environment broadly:

> *...the aggregate of... external conditions... affecting the life... of an organism. It can be divided into physical, biologic, social, cultural; any or all of which can influence the health status of the population.*

While it is true that "external conditions... affecting... life" can be grouped as stated, these conditions can be understood only if the related toxicology is discounted. Yet medicine usually avoids toxicology.

An exceptional WHO document strives to resolve the Germs vs Environment confusion.[9]

> *...definition of environment is... limited to include... only modifiable environmental factors, that is, factors readily amenable to change...*

Excluded are the following items from discussions of "environment".

> *Person-to-person transmission*

> *Biological agents*

---

[9] A Prüss-Ustün et al., *Preventing Disease Through Healthy Environments: A Global Assessment of the Burden of Disease from Environmental Risks* (WHO, 2016), http://www.who.int/quantifying_ehimpacts/publications/preventing-disease/en/.

Environment (my definition)

The WHO document, though good, remains burdened with some political correctness. A better definition would be more direct.

As will be demonstrated, disease is mostly industrial-toxicological. To avoid confusion, germs should be excluded from the definition of environment because germ science is soft and more politicized than toxicology.

Diagnostics are more effective when germs are viewed as toxicological symptoms, micro-ecological imbalances in a symbiotic context. Bad genes and mutations should also be viewed as symptoms.

As will be demonstrated, Modern Medicine does not resolve its contradictions, preferring monopoly silence and bogus stories imbedded in advertising, journalism, science, law and regulations.

Toxicology is empirical and provable, though unfortunately subject to industrial politics. It is nevertheless the best path to understanding pathology.

Consider toxicological causation from the perspective of Hippocrates, "The Father of Modern Medicine", who lived in ancient Greece, 460-370BC. Here is a toxicological slant on two of his pertinent quotes.

For stability, the body resists poisoning until it eventually is overwhelmed and disease appears:

> *Illnesses do not come upon us out of the blue. They are developed from small daily sins against Nature. When enough sins have accumulated, illnesses will suddenly appear.*

Diseases are normal responses to poisoning:

We call them diseases but they are the cure of diseases.

2 | Microcephaly

Key concepts

Microcephaly means "small brain". When this condition is found, it is usually found at birth, and thereby known as "congenital microcephaly". (Congenital means "at birth".)

Wikipedia, a clear representative of Modern Medicine, describes microcephaly.[10]

> *Microcephaly is a medical condition... a smaller than normal head. Often people with the disorder have an intellectual disability, poor motor function, poor speech, abnormal facial features, seizures, and dwarfism.*

[10] *Wikipedia*, "Microcephaly," June 22, 2016, https://en.wikipedia.org/wiki/Microcephaly.

***Wikipedia* hypes genetic causation.**

> *The disorder may stem from a wide variety of conditions that cause abnormal growth of the brain, or from syndromes associated with chromosomal abnormalities... [Genetic] mutation... causes primary microcephaly.*

The epidemic

***Wikipedia* summarizes the epidemic in NE Brazil with a 2015-2016 timeline while hyping Zika virus causation for the epidemic.**

> *The 2015–16 Zika virus epidemic... a widespread epidemic of... fever, caused by the Zika virus, is ongoing in the Americas and the Pacific. The outbreak began in early 2015 in Brazil, then spread to other parts...*
>
> *In February 2016, WHO declared the outbreak a Public Health Emergency of International Concern as evidence grew that Zika can cause birth defects as well as neurological problems...*
>
> *The virus is spread mainly by the Aedes aegypti mosquito.... A number of countries have issued travel warnings...*[11]

The epidemic is real

Many believe the epidemic is not real, saying say it is merely a change in reporting or diagnostic methods, or that it is due to journalistic hype. An example is ECLAMC (12/30/2015):

---

[11] *Wikipedia*, "2015–16 Zika Virus Epidemic," July 8, 2016, https://en.wikipedia.org/wiki/2015%E2%80%9316_Zika_virus_epidemic.

> *The observed excessive number of cases is probably due to active search and over-diagnosis.*[12]

ECLAMC overlooked crucial information, such as the Soares (2016), a WHO Bulletin that precisely reports the epidemic timeline.[13]

Soares (2016)

At the end of 2015, the timeline was constructed. This investigation had been tasked to *The Network*, which is headquartered in Recife, state of Pernambuco, NE Brazil.

The Network is a telemedicine network committed to overseeing clinical work, teaching DUS via live-streaming internet video, bringing DUS expertise to clinicians and facilitating consultations with specialists such as neonatal heart surgeons. It is managed by Dr. Sandra da Silva Mattos.

To determine the microcephaly timeline, newborn head circumferences were determined within the client population served by *The Network* during a four-year period (2012-2015). These measurements were compared against historical documents.

Microcephaly was determined by three different methods, clearly describing an epidemic suddenly emerging in July 2012, and continuing through 2015 and into 2016.

---

[12] "Summary and Conclusion - Zika Virus - Microcephaly," *ECLAMC - Estudio Colaborativo Latino Americano de Malformaciones Congénitas*, December 30, 2015, http://www.eclamc.org/descargas/NS-724-2015_ECLAMC-ZIKA%20VIRUS_V-FINAL_012516.docx.

[13] Juliana Sousa Soares de Araújo et al., "Microcephaly in Northeastern Brazil: A Review of 16 208 Births between 2012 and 2015," *Bulletin of the World Health Organization*, January 29, 2016, doi:10.2471/BLT.16.170639.

Many persons witnessed the epidemic at ground zero.

Dr. Ana van der Linden (WSJ):

> *"With all my years of experience, I **never had seen an epidemic of this magnitude**," said Dr. Ana van der Linden, 75 years old, the matriarch of a family of five physicians....*

Dr. Vanessa van Der Linden (*Time*):

> *Dr Vanessa van der Linden... Recife... was the first person to spot a possible link between the Zika virus and a spike in the increase in microcephaly births... "I saw three cases of microcephaly in one day last August when normally I would see one maybe every three months. **It was very strange**."*[14]

If "three cases... in one day" is a trend then that would be a 270x rise in microcephaly incidence, August 2015.

Dr. Timmerman (WSJ):

> *Dr. Timerman said. "Data in Brazil on this subject is still precarious, but I suspect that the data is being **underestimated** more than overestimated."*[15]

Dr. Angela Rocha, head of the infectious-disease unit Oswaldo Cruz public hospital in Recife in the state of Pernambuco (Sky News):

---

[14] Alex Crawford, "Zika Virus May Have Spread To Common Mosquito," *Sky News*, January 29, 2016, http://news.sky.com/story/zika-virus-may-have-spread-to-common-mosquito-10146129.

[15] Reed Johnson, "The Brazilian Doctors Who Sounded the Alarm on Zika and Microcephaly," *Wall Street Journal*, January 29, 2016, http://graphics.wsj.com/how-zika-spreads/.

> *In 43 years as a doctor, I have seen outbreaks of polio and cholera but never anything **as shocking** as this. The panic, stress and uncertainty of these women, it is difficult to watch.*[16]

By empirical measurement, also, the newborn head circumference (as measured at birth) changed extremely and suddenly. A horrific epidemic undoubtedly emerged.

Causation

Wikipedia lists possible causation agents for microcephaly. The list is useful though misleading. Its four-point outline hypes genetic causation and omits radiation causation. Here are the main categories [my annotations in brackets]:

Isolated [microcephaly alone, as genetically caused]

Syndrome [microcephaly comorbid, as genetic caused]

Acquired [causation by injury, germs, chemicals]

Other [causation by maternal problems]

I assumed *Wikipedia* to be a work in progress, eventually meant to display two category of microcephaly (isolated and syndrome).

I expected that each category would eventually have three subcategories (genetic, acquired, other), as follows.

Isolated microcephaly

Genetic

[16] Matt Sandy, "Worried Mothers Fear for Their Children at Ground Zero of the Zika Outbreak," *Time*, February 1, 2016, http://time.com/4202993/worried-mothers-fear-for-their-children-at-ground-zero-of-the-zika-outbreak/.

Acquired, e.g., injury, germs, chemicals, genetics

Other, e.g., maternal problems

Syndrome [microcephaly comorbid]

Genetic

Acquired, e.g., injury, germs, chemicals, genetics

Other, e.g., maternal problems

To date, *Wikipedia* has not improved. It mostly lists genetic categories and some infection categories. It nearly always faults the patient. Iatrogenia (medico causation) is omitted.

For example, in addition to:

- Genetic [weak ancestors]
- Infection [weak immune system, bad habits]

There is:

- Alcoholic mother [personal weakness].
- Lead poisoning, e.g., paint chips [ignorance or carelessness].
- Radiation [nuclear, Fukushima, Hiroshima, sunshine]

Wikipedia hypes genetic causation despite genetics having the least valid scientific support. (Details later herein and in Part C.)

"Radiation to the mother" is under the category "Other" (as though this were trivial).

Prenatal radiation ("Radiation to the fetus") is omitted despite the obvious hazard.

Reorganizing *Wikipedia's* list

I merged the *Wikipedia* outline with Pilu (1999), keeping *Wikipedia* and Pilu's apparent mainstream intent (to prioritize genetic causation).[17]

Pilu describes causation as

> *Genetic*
>
> *Environmental*
>
> *Unknown*

This view is confirmed by Ashwal (2009), microcephaly with comorbidities ("syndromic"), or isolated ("pure"):

> *Microcephaly may* ***be described as syndromic or as pure,*** *primary, or true (microcephalia vera... These terms do not imply a distinct etiology and [both] can be seen with* ***either genetic or environmental causes*** *of neurodevelopmental impairment.*[18]

---

[17] Gianluigi Pilu, Philippe Jeanty, "Microcephaly," *The Fetus*, July 27, 1999, http://sonoworld.com/fetus/page.aspx?id=127.

[18] Stephen Ashwal et al., "Practice Parameter: Evaluation of the Child with Microcephaly (an Evidence-Based Review)," *Neurology* 73, no. 11 (September 15, 2009): 887–97, doi:10.1212/WNL.0b013e3181b783f7.

Causation graph

See my graphic summary of *Wikipedia*'s causation list by category.

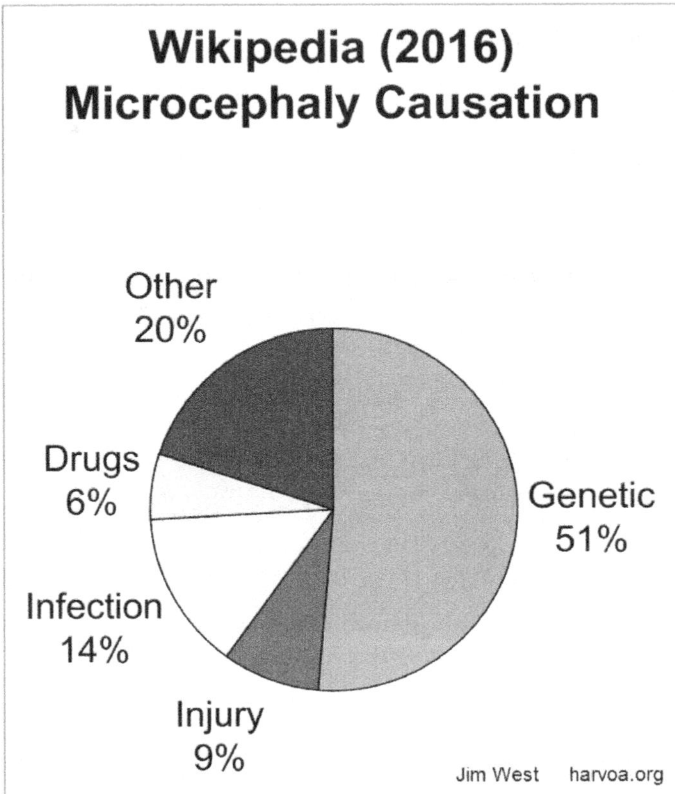

Wikipedia *INVERTED,* corrects industrial bias

Wikipedia is absurd in view of DUS Book 1 ("50 Human Studies..."), where DUS is demonstrated to be hazardous enough to be able to cause microcephaly. Generally, the mainstream allows no possibility for DUS causation for any disease, let alone microcephaly. The word "ultrasound" is excluded from key disease causation literature.

Critical environmental literature (such as my books) generally demonstrates that industrial dominance of medical topics is so complete that it is able to invert public perception, as if disease causation is not industrial.

In a related field (EMF radiation), Henry Lai, PhD found that the results of industry-funded studies are generally the INVERSION of independent studies:

> *When you look at the non-industry sponsored research, it's about three to one-three out of every four papers shows an effect," Lai says. "Then, if you look at the industry-funded research, it's almost opposite — only one out of every four papers shows an effect.*[19]

Thus, with the industrial illusion so complete and predictable, truth can be estimated by simply inverting the industrial view. The reader should ultimately be convinced of this inverted view. See my INVERTED view of the *Wikipedia* pie-graph:

---

[19] Rob Harrill, "Wake Up Call: Cover Stroy," March 2005, https://www.washington.edu/alumni/columns/march05/wakeupcall04.html.

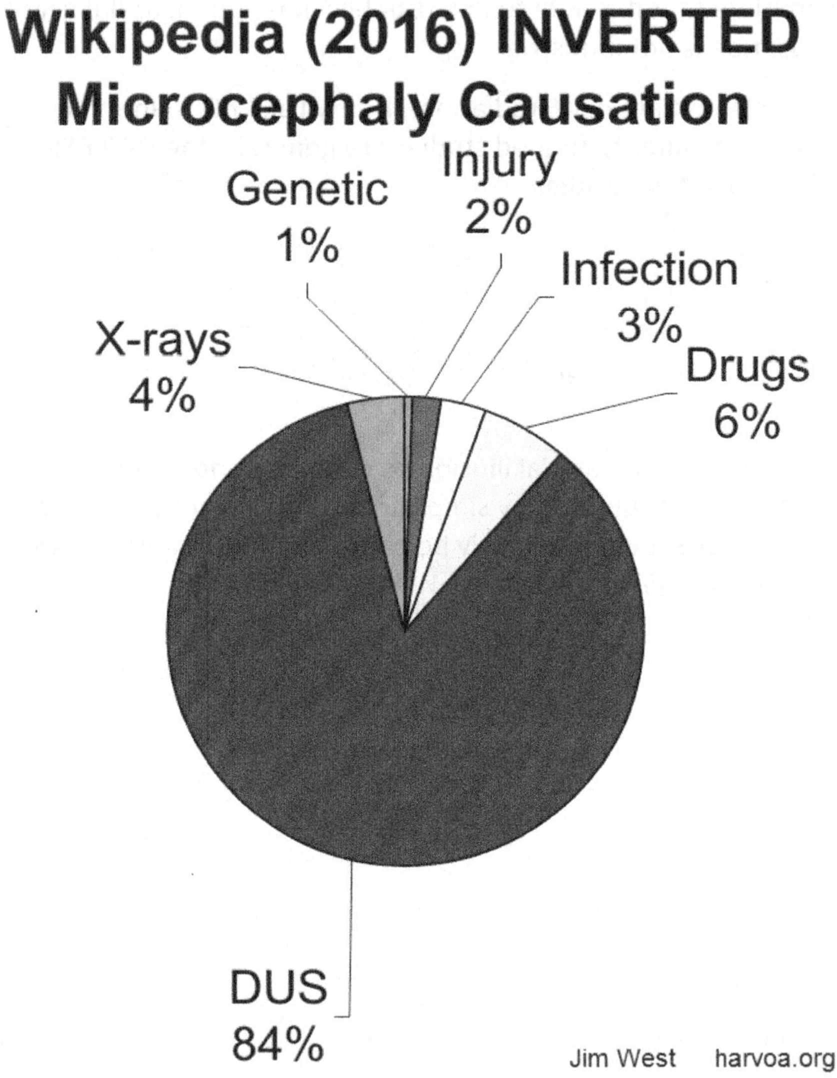
Wikipedia (2016) INVERTED
Microcephaly Causation
Genetic
1%
Injury
2%
Infection
3%
Drugs
6%
X-rays
4%
DUS
84%
Jim West harvoa.org

Genetic causation

Wikipedia:

> *A homozygous mutation in one of* ***the microcephalin genes causes*** *primary microcephaly.*

Wikipedia confidentially uses the word "causes" despite the fact that genetic causation is unproven. The science is associative. The fundamental toxicology has not been discounted. Genetic causation is fake news in a science format. See online the critical work of Jay Joseph, and see further details in Part C.

World Health Organization (WHO)

WHO describes microcephaly.[20]

> *Microcephaly is a condition where a baby is born with a* ***small head*** *or the head stops growing after birth... Babies born with microcephaly* ***may*** *[have or develop neurological and behavioral diseases].*

Dutifully hypes Zika virus causation:

> *The severity of microcephaly ranges from mild to severe. Many babies born with microcephaly may demonstrate no other symptoms at birth but go on to develop epilepsy, cerebral palsy, learning disabilities, hearing loss and vision problems. In some cases, children with microcephaly develop entirely normally.*
>
> *Although not proven, researchers are studying a potential [causative link with]* ***Zika virus infection.***

---

[20] "WHO | Microcephaly [Fact Sheet]," *WHO*, accessed July 13, 2016, http://www.who.int/mediacentre/factsheets/microcephaly/en/.

...Often diagnosis is made at birth or at a later stage.

Describes common causes:

Infections in the womb: toxoplasmosis (caused by a parasite found in undercooked meat), rubella, herpes, syphilis, cytomegalovirus and HIV.

Exposure to toxic chemicals: maternal exposure to heavy metals like arsenic and mercury, alcohol, ***radiation****, and smoking.*

Genetic abnormalities such as Down syndrome.

Severe malnutrition during fetal life.

WHO lists "infections" first, though germ causation is moot because its science fails to discount toxicology.

WHO mentions "radiation" without specifying type, thereby allowing images of the less likely type, nuclear radiation.

Stanford Children's Health (San Francisco, CA)

Here is another microcephaly causation list where the word "radiation" is omitted:

Theories suggest that the following may predispose a fetus to problems that affect the normal development of the head during pregnancy:

Exposure to hazardous chemicals or substances

Methylmercury poisoning

Lack of proper vitamins and nutrients in the diet

Cytomegalovirus, rubella, or varicella infection

Prescription or illegal drug and alcohol consumption

Untreated phenylketonuria

Stanford omits "Radiation" for good reason. It immediately recommends profitable genetic counseling with radiological examinations, "CT-scans", "MRI", and "prenatal ultrasound".[21] It displays no concern for its compounding of toxic radiation exposure.

The Mayo Clinic

The Mayo Clinic is most predictable. It hypes microcephaly causation as Original Sin, i.e., it promotes mutated genes, infection, drugs and alcohol (not "pharmaceuticals"), while omitting "medical radiation".[22]

> *Microcephaly usually is the result of abnormal brain development... Microcephaly may be genetic. Other causes may include:*
>
> *Craniosynostosis. The premature fusing of the joints (sutures) between the bony plates that form an infant's skull...*
>
> *Chromosomal abnormalities...*
>
> *Decreased oxygen to the fetal brain. Certain complications of pregnancy or delivery can impair oxygen delivery to the fetal brain.*

---

[21] Stanford Children's Health, "Microcephaly," accessed February 12, 2016, http://www.stanfordchildrens.org/en/topic/default?id=microcephaly-90-P02610.

[22] "Microcephaly Causes," *Mayo Clinic*, accessed March 16, 2017, http://www.mayoclinic.org/diseases-conditions/microcephaly/basics/causes/con-20034823.

Infections of the fetus...

Exposure to drugs, alcohol or certain toxic chemicals in the womb...

Severe malnutrition...

Uncontrolled phenylketonuria [PKU], in the mother. PKU is a birth defect that hampers the body's ability to break down the amino acid phenylalanine.

Boston Children's Hospital

This Q & A is from the microcephaly webpage of Boston Children's Hospital.[23] The radiation topic is omitted. Patient fault is accented. Germs are blamed.

Question 1*: Is there any way to prevent it [microcephaly]?*

Answer 1*: When microcephaly is genetic... nothing can be done to prevent it.*

If there is no genetic link... expectant mothers can lessen their chances of having a baby with microcephaly by avoiding the following...

use of drugs or alcohol

abuse of prescription medications

poor nutrition

untreated phenylketonuria (PKU)

---

[23] "Microcephaly Symptoms & Causes | Boston Children's Hospital," *Archive.is*, February 25, 2016, http://archive.is/vVKXr.

exposure to certain viruses – especially chickenpox, rubella or cytomegalovirus

exposure to toxic chemicals

[...]

Question 2: Can microcephaly be detected during pregnancy?

*Answer 2: If your child has the congenital form of microcephaly – **meaning it is caused** by an inherited defect in his genes – it might be possible to detect the disorder with a **prenatal ultrasound** during the third trimester of pregnancy.*

Note in Answer 2, where "the congenital form of microcephaly" is completely assigned to "inherited defect in his genes", without any consideration of prenatal toxicology.

Note that DUS radiation is mentioned only as an examination procedure, not as a teratogen (agent of fetal damage).

A new causation *Hypothesis* is necessary.

3 | *The Hypothesis*

Causation assessed

The Hypothesis is multi-facetted with many possible corollaries. It asserts that DUS is the cause of the recent microcephaly epidemic in NE Brazil.

It is outlined here without references.

Given: DUS capability

The Chinese Human Studies (CHS) and earlier Euro-American studies clearly demonstrate the destructive potential of prenatal DUS. It must then be a contender for the dominant cause of microcephaly, present-era.

- DUS directly causes fetal disease.
- DUS is the primary initiator of fetal vulnerabilities

DUS establishes toxic synergies. It establishes vulnerabilities to subsequent stressors: pharmaceuticals (antibiotics, vaccines, drugs), exhaust, pesticides, fracking effluents, EMF, etc.

An exceptional modern Western study is Webb (2016), which indicts prenatal DUS for Autism Spectrum Disorder (ASD) and argues for a stronger adherence to FDA [24] guidelines. Pierre Mourad, PhD, of the University of Washington in Seattle, is lead author.[25] See Appendix B | Webb (2016) and AIUM for the industrial defense, Mourad's reply, and my notes.

Obstacles to investigation

- There are no DUS causation studies for microcephaly from any era.
- Modern Medicine falsely claims there are virtually no modern DUS studies for any disease.
- Modern Medicine does not recognize nor resolve the many studies that indict DUS.
- The word "ultrasound" is missing from key causation literature (any disease).

Many studies indict DUS yet are designed to be inconclusive. Neutering is required for publication. Studies often do not include a zero-exposure "control group", preferring less exposure. Early era studies, before FDA/1991[26], are declared inapplicable to the modern era despite using lower ultrasound intensities than used in the modern era.

---

[24] The Food and Drug Administration.

[25] Sara Jane Webb et al., "Severity of ASD Symptoms and Their Correlation with the Presence of Copy Number Variations and Exposure to First Trimester Ultrasound," *Autism Research*, August 1, 2016, n/a-n/a, doi:10.1002/aur.1690.

[26] FDA/1991 is the acronym for the critical historical DUS date, when FDA raised allowable DUS machine intensities by 8x 15x. Acronym "FDA/1991".

Hormesis is the name of a fundamental dose/response concept that, when ignored or misused, allows scientists to declare their observations insignificant.

My skepticism re medical "science", especially in the field of ultrasound, is supported by comments found in Anderson and Barrett (1979-1981)[27] and recent lectures by James Lyons-Weiler, PhD. Both clearly describe routine corruption.

Over 800 ultrasound studies were conducted before Ellisman (1987) wrote:

> *...reviews of the literature on ultrasound bioeffects... reveal that most studies were inadequately designed...* [28]

As a form of censorship, these obstacles are (to some extent) evidence for DUS causation.

Direct evidence

- The CHS demonstrate DUS causation for the prominent symptoms associated with microcephaly, e.g., brain, eye, and other fetal organ damage. At clinical intensities, DUS can disintegrate cells, DNA, and other macro-molecular complexes.
- CKimmel (1983), mice study, demonstrates DUS causation for growth restriction, brain damage, and general malformations, though it declares its observations inconclusive.

---

[27] D W Anderson and J T Barrett, "Ultrasound: A New Immunosuppressant," *Clinical Immunology and Immunopathology* 14, no. 1 (September 1979): 18–29.

[28] Mark H Ellisman, Darryl Erik Palmer, and Michael P André, "Diagnostic Levels of Ultrasound May Disrupt Myelination," *Experimental Neurology* 98, no. 1 (October 1987): 78–92, doi:10.1016/0014-4886(87)90073-2.

Circumstantial evidence

- Microcephaly is usually comorbid with intrauterine growth restriction (IUGR) syndrome. Ultrasound has been demonstrated causative for IUGR.
- Microcephaly syndrome usually occurs in the womb at approximately 20 weeks gestation. This is also the usual gestation date for DUS exposure.
- X-rays are known to cause microcephaly syndrome. By considering the similarity of X-rays and DUS in terms of dose/response and comorbidity patterns, DUS causation for microcephaly can be inferred.
- A historical precedent exists in medical radiology. Careless prenatal DUS history is similar to the earlier history of careless prenatal X-ray examinations. John Gofman, MD, PhD and others have critically documented X-ray history and causation science, though not in terms of rubella.[29]
- Except for DUS, all other toxic agents, such as X-rays, pharmaceuticals (antibiotics, vaccines, etc.) and pesticides (insecticides, herbicides, larvicides), fail in terms of time, location, and dose.
- Gene causation fails in time and location, and its construct fails fundamentally.
- Zika virus fails in time and location, and its construct fail fundamentally. Other infectious agents either fail in time and location or fail in their fundamental constructs.

---

[29] John W. Gofman, M.D., Ph.D., "Radiation-Inducible Chromosome Injuries: Some Recent Evidence on MAJOR Health Consequences," 1992, https://ratical.org/radiation/CNR/RICI.html.

Strong circumstantial evidence

- Most epidemic cases were newborns served by *The Network*.
- High-exposure prenatal DUS had been applied by *The Network* to all pregnant women within its client population, within the epidemic region of NE Brazil, just 6 months before the epidemic. Generally, routine DUS can begin as early as 3 months gestation. Crosscheck: 6+3 = 9 months (normal gestation period).
- The epidemic and *The Network's* prenatal ultrasound program are both unique yet aligned in time, location, symptoms, and DUS exposure (unique worldwide and in history).

Conclusion

- **The microcephaly epidemic was caused by a unique high-exposure prenatal DUS program within *The Network*.**
- DUS is the major cause of microcephaly in the present era, the primary initiator of most childhood diseases and relevant adult diseases.
- The Zika virus paradigm is an industrial cover for prenatal DUS damage.
- Modern Medicine bias is maniacal, with its evidence for microcephaly causation weak, contradictory and loud.

Corollaries

- There is a historical precedent to the present era of Congenital Zika Syndrome (CZS) cover story. During the earlier X-ray era (before routine DUS, before the late 1970s), the cover story was Congenital Rubella Syndrome (CRS). CZS and CRS are similar syndromes.

- The human papillomavirus (HPV) paradigm for warts is the cover for gynecological DUS damage in young women.
- *The Hypothesis* revolutionizes medicine by giving support to existing toxicology of prenatal radiation. This applies to radiation damage appearing in newborns, then with maturity, children and adults. This applies to both the physiological and psychological fields of medicine.

Other possibilities

The Network may have subjected the pregnant mothers with unusual drugs, CT-scans, or prenatal MRI, but there is no such evidence. Such theories are complex and unlikely.

Appendix A | Proof Tables presents other views of *The Hypothesis.*

The following material supports or employs *The Hypothesis*.

4 | Preliminary Evidence

Circumstantial proof

Most modern DUS studies are empirical investigations of the effects of prenatal DUS within the human womb (*in utero*). Various fetal organs, including the brain, have been studied following abortion. Though these are not studies of microcephaly causation per se, they are closely related to the ideal of a direct study. They directly demonstrate a wide array of DUS damage.

The two dominant mainstream disease paradigms (germs and genes) protect the practice of diagnostic ultrasound, however, such paradigms are almost always based upon circumstantial evidence. Medical science advertises itself as empirical, but in general, that is only superficially true.

Virus causation

This book's title allows the implication that ultrasound causes Zika virus, but ultrasound actually causes symptoms that are falsely interpreted by the mainstream as a virus.

Virology is technically sophisticated, but the science is associative and indirect. *Field's Virology* (1990) represents a century of medical science:

> *The problem [of causation] is... difficult... virologists have had to evaluate causation indirectly via "guilt by association"...*[30]

Worse than that, there is generally no evidence for the existence of any virus with which to associate "guilt". For example, the famous studies of poliovirus isolation have been deflated by Howard Urnovitz, PhD, with journalist Neenyah Ostrom.[31] In Australia, The Perth Group reveals the vacuity of HIV (virus) fundamentals.[32] Perth deconstructs HIV (virus) paradigm only, not wanting to appear radical, however, the principles of Perth's critique can be applied to any supposed virus. Standing monetary awards, such as those offered by biochemist Stefan Lanka, are available to anyone who can prove causation for various viruses.[33,34]

---

[30] "Virus Taxonomy," in *Fields' Virology*, vol. 1 (Lippincott Williams & Wilkins, 1990).

[31] Neenyah Ostrom and Howard Urnovitz, PhD, "Will The Poliovirus Eradication Program Rid the World of Childhood Paralysis?," n.d., http://harvoa.org/polio/misc/OstromParalyticpolio.htm.

[32] www.ThePerthGroup.com

[33] "HIV & AIDS - VirusMyth AIDS WebSite - Missing Virus Award," accessed July 27, 2017, http://www.virusmyth.com/aids/award.htm.

[34] Paul Fassa, "German Supreme Court Upholds Biologist's Claim That Measles Virus Does Not Exist," March 5, 2017, http://vaccineimpact.com/2017/german-supreme-court-upholds-biologists-claim-that-measles-virus-does-not-exist/.

Irrefutable: Virology is moot because it never discounts even the most obvious toxicology.[35] Virologists do not debate their positions in public as they would have nothing to gain and everything to lose.

The reader should resolve any doubts by way of the aforesaid references, as this book accordingly dismisses virus theories. This is not an arrogant dismissal as the reader will find.

The mainstream dramatization of germ theory and the illusions of infection are discussed with a dash of humor in the Appendix C | Infectious Illusions. Zika virus is deconstructed in detail in Part B.

Genetic causation

Genetic causation science is admittedly "associative" according to the authoritative genetic pathology text, Kohn (2003). Note that MZ means "monozygote" (genetic twin), and DZ means "dizygote" (fraternal twin):

> *Twin studies are the* ***gold standard****... on... genetic etiology [causation]...* ***Researchers assume*** *that MZ and DZ twins are similar [re] shared environment... The* ***only way to overcome this limitation*** *is by comparing concordance rates of MZ twins who were reared together or apart... quite impractical for genetic research. Nevertheless, twin studies are considered the best estimate of heritability...*[36]

However, it is worse than Kohn admits. The environmental influence on even the emergence of MZ vs DZ twins is not understood nor discounted.

---

[35] Jim West, "Pesticides and Polio," *The Townsend Letter for Doctors and Patients*, June 2000.

[36] Yoav Kohn and Bernard Lerer, "Chapter 2: Methodological Advances in Psychiatric Genetics," in *Handbook of Medical Psychiatry* (CRC Press, 2003).

And even worse, the environmental influence on the emergence of twins themselves is not understood nor discounted.

So goes the "gold standard" of genetic causation science. (Details in Part C.)

ZIKA SCIENCE

CDC (Center for Disease Control and Prevention), WHO (World Health Organization), *The New York Times, The Washington Post,* etc. promote Zika virus causation for the epidemic.

Rasmussen (2016)[37] is cited as an authoritative overview, yet it misrepresents the science fundamentals.

Timeline fails

Rasmussen paints an epidemic timeline that is three years too late in its attempt to associate Zika virus discovery in Brazil with the emergence of the epidemic in Brazil:

> *Since the identification of the Zika virus in Brazil* ***in early 2015****, the virus has spread rapidly... An increase in the number of infants with* ***microcephaly in Brazil was first noted in September 2015,*** *after the recognition of Zika virus transmission in the country earlier in the year.*

The epidemic actually began in 2012 with scientists finding not Zika, but rubella and herpes "virus infections" in nearly all microcephaly cases.

Remember that the aforesaid *Wikipedia* section also uses the false 2015 timeline.

---

[37] Sonja A. Rasmussen et al., "Zika Virus and Birth Defects — Reviewing the Evidence for Causality," *New England Journal of Medicine* 374, no. 20 (May 19, 2016): 1981–87, doi:10.1056/NEJMsr1604338.

Zika fundamentals fail

Despite the hype, most scientists agree that there is no conclusive evidence for Zika virus causation. Some scientists politely argue against Zika virus. Lay critics find the virus a blatant hoax, with myself and others having critically reviewed the study that claims discovery of the virus in 1947. (Details in Part C.)

Mainstream Zika virus studies actually disprove causation, yet are spun to support causation.

Rasmussen convicts Zika virus while admitting that no laboratory study demonstrates microcephaly causation. It brings a dubious epidemiological association. It even misrepresents weak mainstream criterion in its efforts to convict the virus. It does not verify the fundamental existence of this virus.

Cugola (2016)[38] infected mice with a "Zika virus" to demonstrate microcephaly causation, yet no microcephaly resulted. Intrauterine Growth Restriction (IUGR) was found and a causation rationale spun for microcephaly virus causation, spun on the basis that IUGR and microcephaly are usually comorbid. Nevertheless, only "signs of microcephaly" were found by Cugola. These were biochemical, hormonal and microbiological effects, not microcephaly itself.

Cugola's observations (not its conclusions) actually reject Zika virus causation. Microcephaly was not observed from "Zika virus" exposure. IUGR was observed but not microcephaly. The impact of these observations cannot be admitted, as that would be heresy, so the study spins itself 180 degrees as supposed evidence for Zika virus causation.

---

[38] Fernanda R. Cugola et al., "The Brazilian Zika Virus Strain Causes Birth Defects in Experimental Models," *Nature* advance online publication (May 11, 2016), doi:10.1038/nature18296.

IUGR and GADD45a

GADD45a is the acronym for the Growth Arrest and DNA Damage gene. Upon exposure to environmental stress, this gene increases its expression of specific proteins[39] as a natural protective response.[40]

Contradiction re "hallmark"

X-rays are known to cause IUGR and to increase GADD45a expression of stress response proteins. This is "up-regulation".

GADD45a up-regulation is referred to as "the hallmark of ionizing radiation".[41] (Ionizing radiation is any radiation type that, while disrupting matter, can create ion pairs. Examples of ionizing radiation are the higher frequency types of ultraviolet light, X-rays, and gamma radiation.)

However, DUS can also cause GADD45a up-regulation, and DUS is non-ionizing radiation.[42] Thus up-regulation cannot actually be the "hallmark of ionizing radiation".

---

[39] Jeffrey Hildesheim et al., "Gadd45a Protects against UV Irradiation-Induced Skin Tumors, and Promotes Apoptosis and Stress Signaling via MAPK and p53," *Cancer Research* 62, no. 24 (December 15, 2002): 7305–15.

[40] Biji Mathew et al., "Role of GADD45a in Murine Models of Radiation- and Bleomycin-Induced Lung Injury," *American Journal of Physiology - Lung Cellular and Molecular Physiology* 309, no. 12 (December 15, 2015): L1420–29, doi:10.1152/ajplung.00146.2014.

[41] Helen Budworth et al., "DNA Repair and Cell Cycle Biomarkers of Radiation Exposure and Inflammation Stress in Human Blood," *PLOS ONE* 7, no. 11 (November 7, 2012): e48619, doi:10.1371/journal.pone.0048619.

[42] Zvonko Hočevar et al., "Gene Expression Profiling of Rat Fetuses Exposed to 2-Dimensional Ultrasound," *Journal of Ultrasound in Medicine* 31, no. 6 (June 1, 2012): 923–32.

The damaging aspects of DUS radiation are analogous to ionizing radiation and possibly worse.

Consider "down-regulation"

While ultrasound causes up-regulation of GADD45a at certain frequencies, Cugola (2016) found down-regulation (suppression) of GADD45a as a response to its exposure of mice to the so-called Zika virus strain.

> *GADD45a [was] highly suppressed.*

Down-regulation (suppression) of GADD45a gene expression in a mice study makes sense in terms of ultrasound causation within the human epidemic.

"Zika virus strain" cannot be the actual causative agent. It is an extract of hormonal matter and debris from "Zika virus" infected humans, though actually from ultrasound damage. Ultrasound damage causes up-regulation of GADD45a, other stress response products and microbiological debris.

If the extract (the "strain") were injected into mice, as Cugola did, then any normal expression of GADD45a would be suppressed by the presence of competing stress response products in the "strain".

The mainstream would say, "Zika virus just functions that way. It tricks the biological system." This is the usual description of the means by which viruses survive, that they "trick" cells into working for them.

But Zika can only trick the reader. As mentioned, the virus has never been proven to be anything more than a laboratory artifact, i.e., a processed extract of inflammatory matter and cellular debris. Electron microphotographs exist of purported "virus" particles but the particles are not properly characterized (not isolated) nor are they correlated with actual disease symptoms. The virus is a symptom, not a cause nor a germ. It is a biological response to environmental stress, detected in a lab as a chemical that is interpreted as a scary particle germ. (Zika-specific details later.)

Vaccines fail

Vaccine causation theory is promoted by, for example, Viera Scheibner, PhD (a respected authority among anti-vaccinationists).

> *...Sao Paulo announced a mandatory vaccination of pregnant women between the 27th and 36th week of pregnancy, from December 2014 with TDaP vaccine. From early May 2015 a great number of babies were born with microcephaly.*[43]

Contradictory start dates

Vaccine causation theories are based on an epidemic start date of mid-2015.

The epidemic actually began 3 years earlier, in mid-2012.

Thus the vaccine theory fails in time.

Contradictory location

Scheibner wrote:

> *Most of the cases occurred in Pernambuco where most of TDaP vaccines were distributed.*

---

[43] Viera Scheibner, PhD, "Microcephaly in Brazilian Babies: Could Maternal Fever Be a Major Contributing Factor?," *The BMJ*, February 3, 2016, http://www.bmj.com/content/352/bmj.i657/rr-0.

Scheibner's source is Marco Cáceres who wrote of a nation-wide vaccine mandate with the epidemic cases "occurring... notably in the state of Pernambuco":

> *A large portion of these pregnancies are occurring in Brazil's northeastern region, notably in the state of Pernambuco...*

The word "notably" does not confer any special relation. The vaccine theory fails in location because the vaccine mandate was nation-wide, yet the epidemic was mainly limited to *The Network*, of which its membership mainly spanned Pernambuco and Paraíba and to a lesser extent, other nearby states.

Contradictory gestation period

Scheibner wrote:

> *The gestation weeks for the vaccine contradict the "infection" period, which is primarily during the 20th week.*

Cáceres similarly wrote:

> *The CVE report recommended the TDaP vaccine be given to women between the 27th week and 36th week of their pregnancy...*

Zika "virus infection" was found to be a causative risk for microcephaly when it occurs near the 20th week of gestation or earlier, per Brasil (2016). TDaP, however, was mandated between the "27th week and 36th week", i.e., much later, according to Cáceres. Thus, the vaccine theory fails in terms of gestation weeks.

The vaccine theory fails as primary cause, but could possibly have been a contributing cause (as a toxic synergist following DUS) for certain aspects of the epidemic timeline (details in Part B).

Chemicals fail

Environmentalists suspect chemical pollution, at least as a contributing factor, e.g., pesticides, pharmaceuticals, food, water and air pollution. Evidence for direct causation is weak because these agents were present as usual before the epidemic, i.e., they can only be general background contributors to microcephaly causation. No chemical of sufficient toxicity increased beyond its usual background presence in a timely manner to account for the emergence of the epidemic. Chemical agents are not pertinent in time and location.

Pesticides fail

There is no evidence for unusually hazardous pesticide programs that would correlate in time and location.

Larvicide fails

Environmentalists declared the larvicide, Pyriproxyfen, as causative for the microcephaly epidemic, yet Pyriproxyfen could not be sufficient a hazard to have caused the microcephaly epidemic and its presence in time and location do not support causation.

Pyriproxyfen was accused by a non-descript group in Argentina, "Doctors of Crop-Sprayed Towns".

http://ecowatch.com/2016/02/12/larvicide-cause-not-zika/

http://www.gmwatch.org/news/latest-news/16706-argentine-and-brazilian-doctors-name-larvicide-as-potential-cause-of-microcephaly

The claims appear to originate from the following document, which does not bother to reference its claim, "teratogenic".

http://www.reduas.com.ar/wp-content/uploads/downloads/2016/02/Informe-Zika-de-Reduas_TRAD.pdf

I evaluated the toxicity of Pyriproxyfen in drinking water and determined that it would take 16 years of exposure for minimal biological effects to be observed. See the number crunch in Appendix D | Pyriproxyfen.

The larvicide theory was portrayed by *The New York Times* as an example of how absurd science can be if it does not support Zika Virus causation.[44]

Genetics fail

Lyons-Weiler (3/2016)[45] evaluated all of the causation theories for the epidemic (germ, gene, chemical, vaccine, pesticide, and pharmaceutical theories). These were determined to be weak or inconclusive. Strong potential was given to hybrid virus-environmental-genetic theories. Medical radiation was omitted without comment.

DUS causation succeeds

DUS radiation is the most common and well-documented fetal poison, being teratogenic and mutagenic, yet DUS causation studies for microcephaly are missing.

---

[44] Andrew Jacobs, "Conspiracy Theories About Zika Spread Through Brazil With the Virus," *The New York Times*, February 16, 2016, sec. Americas, https://www.nytimes.com/2016/02/17/world/americas/conspiracy-theories-about-zika-spread-along-with-the-virus.html.

[45] James Lyons-Weiler et al., "Areas of Research and Preliminary Evidence on Microcephaly, Guillain-Barré Syndrome and Zika Virus Infection in the Western Hemisphere," *PLOS One*, March 2016.

5 | Teratogens and Mutagens

Causative agents for microcephaly

DEFINITIONS PARAPHRASED FROM BORNER (2008).[46]

Teratogens are agents that cause structural abnormality of the ova, embryo or fetus.

Mutagens are agents that cause genetic mutations or change the frequency of mutations.

Only when an agent causes ***heritable*** genetic effects, is it called a **mutagen**. 90% of mutagens are carcinogenic. Note that "heritable" often refers to effects passed through generations of cells, i.e., observed through cell division (mitosis) in a laboratory environment, in cellular studies.

If the agent causes non-heritable genetic effects, it is called **genotoxic**, and if the agent causes cancer, it is called a **carcinogen**.

---

[46] Alan Borner, "Mutagens, Teratogens and Carcinogens," *EHS Publishing*, December 28, 2008, http://www.ehspublishing.com/index.php?option=com_content&view=article&id=78.

Borner makes an unusual statement that supports radiation causation and challenges chemical and germ causation:

> *Few chemicals are known to be human teratogens...*
>
> *physical factors as ionizing radiation also may cause malformations. X-rays, for example, are potent mutagens and teratogens...*
>
> *On the other hand, viruses or chemicals must be able to cross the placental barrier.*

Teratogens and mutagens can cause microcephaly. Medical radiation can be both teratogenic and mutagenic.

Microcephaly is a "disorder" or "condition". It is not usually discovered before birth. In severe cases, the top of the newborn's skull appears to be missing, as if the top of the head begins just above the eye.

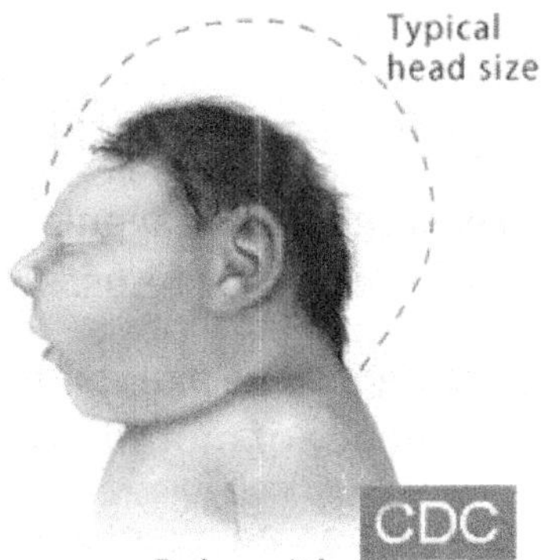

Baby with Severe Microcephaly

The CDC portrays a severe microcephalic child with the apparent visual condition, "squint", one of its common associated symptoms.

Critical exposition

X-rays are a known cause of microcephaly, yet this topic is played down. Anything related to the term, "medical radiation", is entirely omitted from the literature of the Brazil epidemic, and that includes DUS.

Zika virus causation dominates the public view.

Soares (2016) puts on a show of objective humility as it states that ***medical causation*** is more likely than Zika virus:

> *Many other potential factors need to be considered as the cause of the outbreak... teratogens exposure, such as vaccines or drugs used in early pregnancy...*[47]

Soares humbly admits everything but the most obvious (medical radiation).

CHUNG (2005)

Chung (2005)[48] promotes the mainstream view of teratogens that omits DUS and minimizes X-rays. See my graphic rendition of Chung.

---

[47] Soares de Araújo et al., "Microcephaly in Northeastern Brazil."

[48] Wendy Chung, M.D. Ph.D., "Teratogens and Their Effects," in *The New Public Health: An Introduction for the 21st Century*, Theodore H. Tulchinsky; Elena A. Varavikova, editors (Columbia University Press, 2004), http://www.columbia.edu/itc/hs/medical/humandev/2004/Chpt23-Teratogens.pdf.

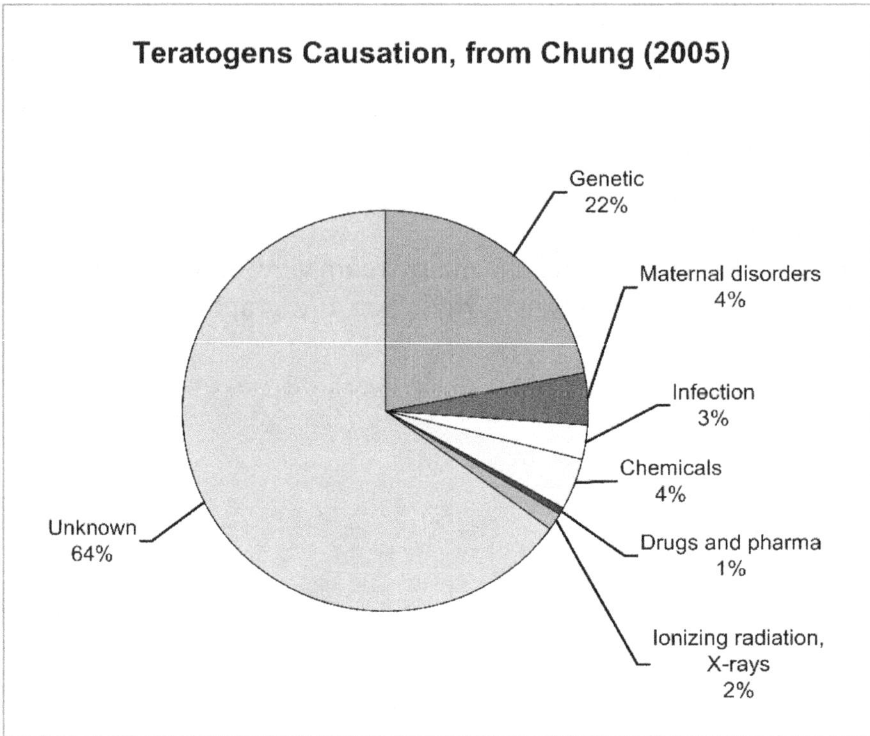

This pie-graph is mainstream reality. It represents the political limits to which monopoly industry can bury environmental reality.

Again consider the work of Henry Lai, PhD where it describes the present industrial inversion of toxicological reality.

By again acknowledging industrial dominance, this time within Chung, I let this representative of industry do the heavy math, then invert Chung's values to obtain a more sensible estimate of reality. Hint: The "Unknown" pie slice would be "X-rays and DUS".

Is inverting Chung too speculative?

- Not if virus and genetic science is critically understood.

- Not if the destructive hazards of DUS are understood.

As stated by Ashwal (2009),

> ***Microcephaly may result from any insult that disturbs early brain growth...***

If there is any doubt that ultrasound can "disturb early brain growth", see DUS Book 1 and herein, see Appendix E | Ultrasound

— Comorbidity —

6 | Growth Restriction

Damage patterns

The epidemic in NE Brazil is not a microcephaly epidemic. It is an epidemic of random fetal damage with infinite variations. Patterns of predominant damage (such as microcephaly) can be characterized.

COMORBIDITY

Comorbidity patterns describe the actual epidemic, i.e., the occurrence of multiple diseases in the same case.

DUS causation can be argued by comparing microcephaly comorbidity patterns with radiation comorbidity patterns.

Cugola (2016) used its observations of growth restriction (IUGR) in mice to argue for Zika virus causation of microcephaly, because IUGR and microcephaly are usually comorbid. Cugola's argument, however, is even more effective when arguing medical radiation causation.

Growth Restriction and Radiation

Schaefer (2001)[49] describes microcephaly and growth restriction as manifestations of medical radiation:

> *The cardinal manifestation of **intrauterine radiation** effects in humans are **growth retardation** and defect of the central nervous system, **mainly microcephaly** with mental retardation and eye malformations...*

Implies a termination protocol:

> *Radiographs outside the genital region and the uterus do not require a **termination** of pregnancy...*

The use of the word "radiographs" by convention refers to X-rays. Yet the etymology of the word indicates it should include both X-ray and DUS images.

Dekaban (1968) describes the early history of frequent fetal X-ray damage.

> *During the 1920s and early 1930s ionizing radiation was widely used... On occasions, the pelvic region was heavily irradiated in [pregnant] women... It was soon learned that irradiation leads to severe damage of the fetus... microcephaly, mental retardation, microphthalmus and cataracts.*
>
> *Since the 1940's, publications on irradiation injury to the human fetus have become less frequent...*[50]

---

[49] Christof Schaefer, *Drugs During Pregnancy and Lactation: Handbook of Prescription Drugs and Comparative Risk Assessment* (Gulf Professional Publishing, 2001), 100–101.

[50] A. S. Dekaban, "Abnormalities in Children Exposed to X-Radiation during Various Stages of Gestation: Tentative Timetable of Radiation Injury to the

As of 1941, such syndromes were being officially ascribed to "rubella", a so-called infectious disease like measles, mild to the adult or child, yet devastating to the newborn.

An obituary of Dr. Alice Stewart, the researcher who did much to document the hazards of prenatal X-rays, describes fetal X-ray radiation through the 1950s. *The New York Times*, 2002:

> *It was an increasingly common practice in the 1950's to X-ray the abdomens of pregnant women to determine the position of their babies...*[51]

Another obituary of Stewart describes the era of prenatal X-rays diminished substantially by mid-1970s. *Telegraph UK* (2002):

> *But by the mid-1970's, other scientists had duplicated [Stewart's] findings on prenatal X-rays, and the practice ended.*
>
> *A single [prenatal] X-ray, well within official safety limits, was enough to double the risk of early cancer, they concluded...*
>
> *[Stewart re censorship:] "Everyone in America who took our side lost their funding... They don't burn you at the stake any more, but they do the equivalent..."*[52]

Human Fetus. I," *Journal of Nuclear Medicine: Official Publication, Society of Nuclear Medicine* 9, no. 9 (September 1968): 471–77.

[51] Carmel McCoubrey, "Alice Stewart, 95; Linked X-Rays to Diseases," *The New York Times*, July 4, 2002, sec. World, https://www.nytimes.com/2002/07/04/world/alice-stewart-95-linked-x-rays-to-diseases.html.

[52] The Telegraph (UK), "Alice Stewart [Eulogy]," August 15, 2002, http://www.telegraph.co.uk/news/obituaries/1404528/Alice-Stewart.html.

Nobody mentions that DUS began to replace prenatal X-rays during this era.

DUS and X-rays

DUS is radiation, governed by hospital Radiology Departments like X-ray imaging. When marketing DUS to patients, the word "radiation" is omitted or the fact denied.

Stevenson (2005) broadens the range of causation:

> *"**Anything that impairs** growth and integrity of the brain from the time of its early development to the end of the postnatal growth period **may lead to microcephaly**."*

In view of the CHS etc., "anything that impairs" must include DUS.

Brasil (2016) places microcephaly within growth restriction syndrome while describing the great microcephaly epidemic:

> *Microcephaly in our cohort was mainly part of an overall composite of restricted fetal growth and not an... isolated finding... other findings such as cerebral calcifications and intrauterine growth restriction were frequently present.*[53]

Rettner (2016) found growth restriction comorbid with microcephaly:

> *[12%] of the Zika-infected women **had fetuses with microcephaly**, but in most of these cases, the fetus also had a condition called **intrauterine growth restriction**, meaning*

---

[53] Patrícia Brasil et al., "Zika Virus Infection in Pregnant Women in Rio de Janeiro — Preliminary Report," *New England Journal of Medicine* 0, no. 0 (March 4, 2016): null, doi:10.1056/NEJMoa1602412.

> *the whole fetus, and not just the head, was abnormally small.*[54]

Growth restriction is a response to damage, for example, damage to cells, hormones, enzymes and DNA. Stressed and damaged by radiation, growth by cell division cannot continue normally. Cell functions and ultrafine structures are most vulnerable to radiation during cell division. A defense is to shut down growth and proceed slowly if at all. In some cases, the mother might be fortunate to miscarriage.

Ocular damage

In NE Brazil, the comorbidities of "Zika virus" microcephaly include ocular damage:

> *"We have seen over 200 children with microcephaly, from which over 40 percent of the confirmed Zika cases have* ***severe ocular lesions,*** *" said Rubens Belfort, Jr., M.D., Ph.D., head professor of ophthalmology at the Federal University of Sao Paulo in Brazil.*[55]

DUS can readily damage the fetal eye. The CHS eye studies advise dwell time at under one minute, having found damage at exposures comparable to that used in NE Brazil.

---

[54] Rachael Rettner and Karen Rowan, "Zika Virus: Microcephaly May Be 'Tip of the Iceberg' for Infant Problems," *Live Science*, March 4, 2016, http://www.livescience.com/53949-zika-virus-fetal-abnormalities.html.

[55] "Studies Show Zika Virus May Cause More Serious Eye Damage in Babies Than Thought," *American Academy of Ophthalmology*, May 31, 2016, http://www.aao.org/eye-health/news/studies-show-zika-virus-may-cause-more-serious-eye.

Hearing damage

The CHS did not specifically study hearing disorders, but it supplied enough observations of various organ damage to allow the inference.

Heart disorders

The CHS did not specifically study heart disorders, but it supplied enough observations of various organ damage to allow the inference.

The Network strongly promoted prenatal echocardiography, i.e., high exposure DUS of the fetal heart.

Preeclampsia

Preeclampsia is often comorbid with microcephaly. It is a complication of pregnancy characterized by high blood pressure, kidney damage, abnormal formation of blood vessels in the placenta and other factors.

McElrath (2010):

> *...fetal* ***growth restriction and preeclampsia*** *are among the strongest correlates of* microcephaly*...*[56]

The CHS found various organ and placental damage at low exposure DUS.

---

[56] Thomas F. McElrath et al., "Factors Associated with Small Head Circumference at Birth among Infants Born before the 28th Week," *American Journal of Obstetrics and Gynecology* 203, no. 2 (August 2010): 138.e1-138.e8, doi:10.1016/j.ajog.2010.05.006.

Mayo Clinic (2016):

> ***Preeclampsia*** *usually begins after* ***20 weeks*** *of pregnancy...*[57]

What else "usually begins after 20 weeks of pregnancy"?

- DUS examinations, usually at the 20th week.
- Growth-restriction.
- Initiation of autism-related damage.
- "Zika virus" or "rubella virus" infection.

Brasil (2016) discusses the timing of fetal Central Nervous System (CNS) disease:

> ***Fetuses infected in the first trimester*** *had findings suggestive of pathologic change during embryogenesis, but Central Nervous System (CNS) abnormalities were also seen in fetuses* ***infected as late as 27 weeks*** *of gestation.* [58]

The gestation timeline for purported Zika virus infection mirrors the common DUS schedule for pregnant women. "Infection" is known to occur mainly during the early 2nd trimester, which just happens to concur with the common ultrasound schedule.

The ability of DUS to cause growth restriction and DNA damage has been demonstrated by Hočevar (2012), JZhang (2002), O'Brien (1976, 1983), the CHS, etc.

---

[57] Mayo Clinic, "Preeclampsia," 2016, http://www.mayoclinic.org/diseases-conditions/preeclampsia/basics/definition/con-20031644.

[58] Brasil et al., "Zika Virus Infection in Pregnant Women in Rio de Janeiro — Preliminary Report."

Prenatal DUS usually occurs during the early 2nd trimester (13th through 26th week of gestation week), as does so-called Zika virus infection. Panchaud (2016):

> *Microcephaly can be caused by several factors leading to brain injury... [because the] majority of neurons are generated* ***prior to 21 weeks gestation****... [when they are most vulnerable.]*

Preeclampsia indicates other possible diagnoses, e.g., Group B Strep (GBS) infection, Zika virus infection, and chorioamnionitis, which bring hazardous antibiotic treatments and further complications.

Infection as DUS exposure

In terms of fetal vulnerability to DUS, the third trimester represents the least risk exposure. This is identical to so-called Zika virus infection, where 3rd trimester is described as least risk.

The gestational timeline for *The Network's* echocardiography is identical to the Zika "virus" infection timeline. Echocardiography is optimally applied during the early 2nd trimester:

> *The optimal timing for performance of a comprehensive transabdominal fetal echocardiogram is 18 to 22 weeks gestation.*[59]

At 20 weeks gestation, medicos may also advocate a higher exposure detailed body scan, i.e., "Level-2 Ultrasound":

---

[59] Jack Rychik, MD, et al, "American Society of Echocardiography Guidelines and Standards for Performance of the Fetal Echocardiogram," 2004.

> *...can take 30 to 45 minutes (depending on how cooperative your little one wants to be).*[60]

Operator guidelines have always advised against first trimester DUS. This has long been ignored, testing the depths of carelessness, incompetence and gullibility.

See my graphic rendering of Zika virus infection and gestation time lines from Brasil (2016). My annotation (blue) indicates the typical DUS date range.

The graph is another example of how Zika virus literature makes better sense if the reader substitutes the term "Zika infection" with "DUS damage".

---

[60] "Level 2 Ultrasound Anatomy Scan | What to Expect," *Whattoexpect*, accessed March 14, 2017, http://www.whattoexpect.com/pregnancy/pregnancy-health/prenatal-testing/ultrasound-anatomy-two.aspx.

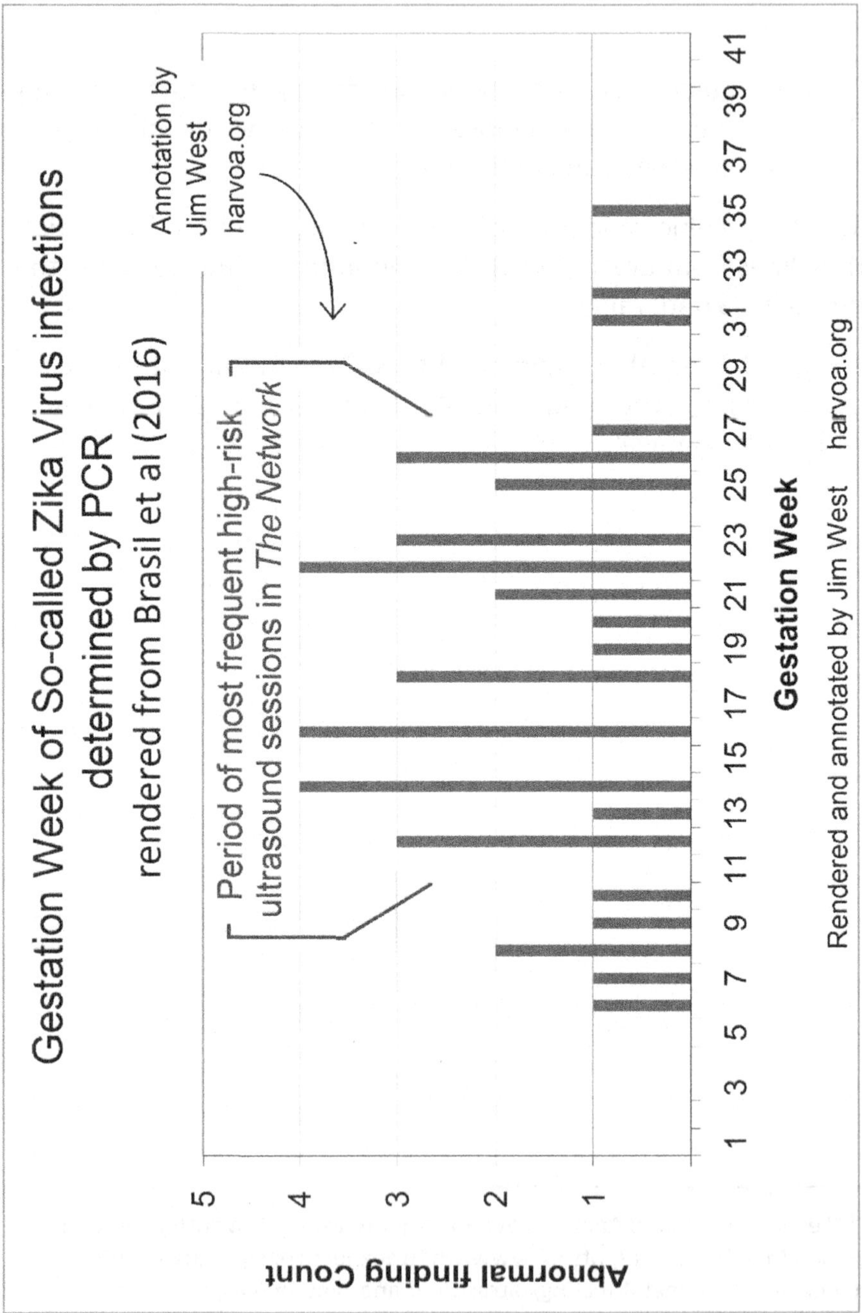
Gestation Week of So-called Zika Virus infections
determined by PCR
rendered from Brasil et al (2016)
Period of most frequent high-risk
ultrasound sessions in *The Network*
Annotation by
Jim West
harvoa.org
Abnormal finding Count
5
4
3
2
1
1 3 5 7 9 11 13 15 17 19 21 23 25 27 29 31 33 35 37 39 41
Gestation Week
Rendered and annotated by Jim West harvoa.org

Weight reduction

Fetal weight reduction is shown from 1990 to 2005 in the next graph. Weight reduction correlates inversely with increasing DUS

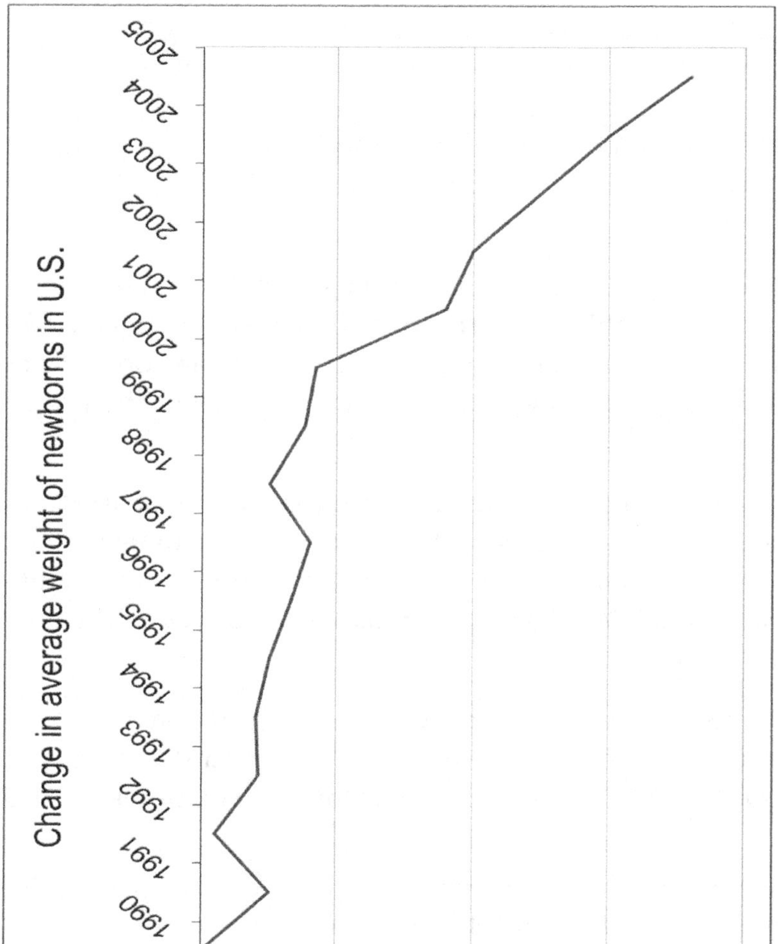

exposure since FDA/1991. The graph was rendered from data presented in an article by Shirley Wang in *The Wall Street Journal* (1/22/2010).[61]

This view is confirmed in Donahue (1996):

> *In 2005, compared with 1990,* **we observed decreases** *in birth weight (−52 grams in the overall population, −79 grams in a homogenous low-risk subgroup) and large for gestational age birth (−1.4% overall, −2.2% in the homogenous subgroup) that were steeper after 1999 and persisted.*[62]

Donahue's stated reduction, ranging from "-52 grams" to "-79 grams", reasonably compares to the findings of Newnham (1993), which found a 25 gram average reduction per newborn in its population study using lower intensity DUS, typical of the pre-1991 era.

The graph correlates with increasing incidence of IUGR since 1991. In a sense, it describes the entire syndrome timeline, including ADHD, autism, hearing, vision, heart disorders, cancer, microcephaly, MACROcephaly (large brain). (MACROcephaly is capitalized for clarity.)

The growth reduction timeline correlates inversely with the explosive rise of the medical industrial administrative class beginning in 1991. DUS is at the core of this growth, providing digital

---

[61] Shirley S. Wang, "Birth Weights Fell From 1990 to 2005," *Wall Street Journal*, January 22, 2010, sec. US, http://www.wsj.com/articles/SB10001424052748704423204575017471267586344.

[62] Sara M. A. Donahue et al., "Trends in Birth Weight and Gestational Length Among Singleton Term Births in the United States," *Obstetrics and Gynecology* 115, no. 2 Pt 1 (February 2010): 357–64, doi:10.1097/AOG.0b013e3181cbd5f5.

diagnostic documentation that is computer and internet friendly. This admin class interfaces throughout the medical-military industrial complex, with government, lobbyists, legislators, lawyers, advertisers, journalists, media, manufacturers, distributors, regulators, and insurance industry.

See graph by Physicians for a National Health Program, used with permission and modified to fit, with my "1991 onward" annotation added.[63]

[63] Judy, "The Rise of the Medical Bureaucrat and Centralized Health Care," Text, *Mises Institute*, (July 13, 2015), https://mises.org/library/rise-medical-bureaucrat-and-centralized-health-care.

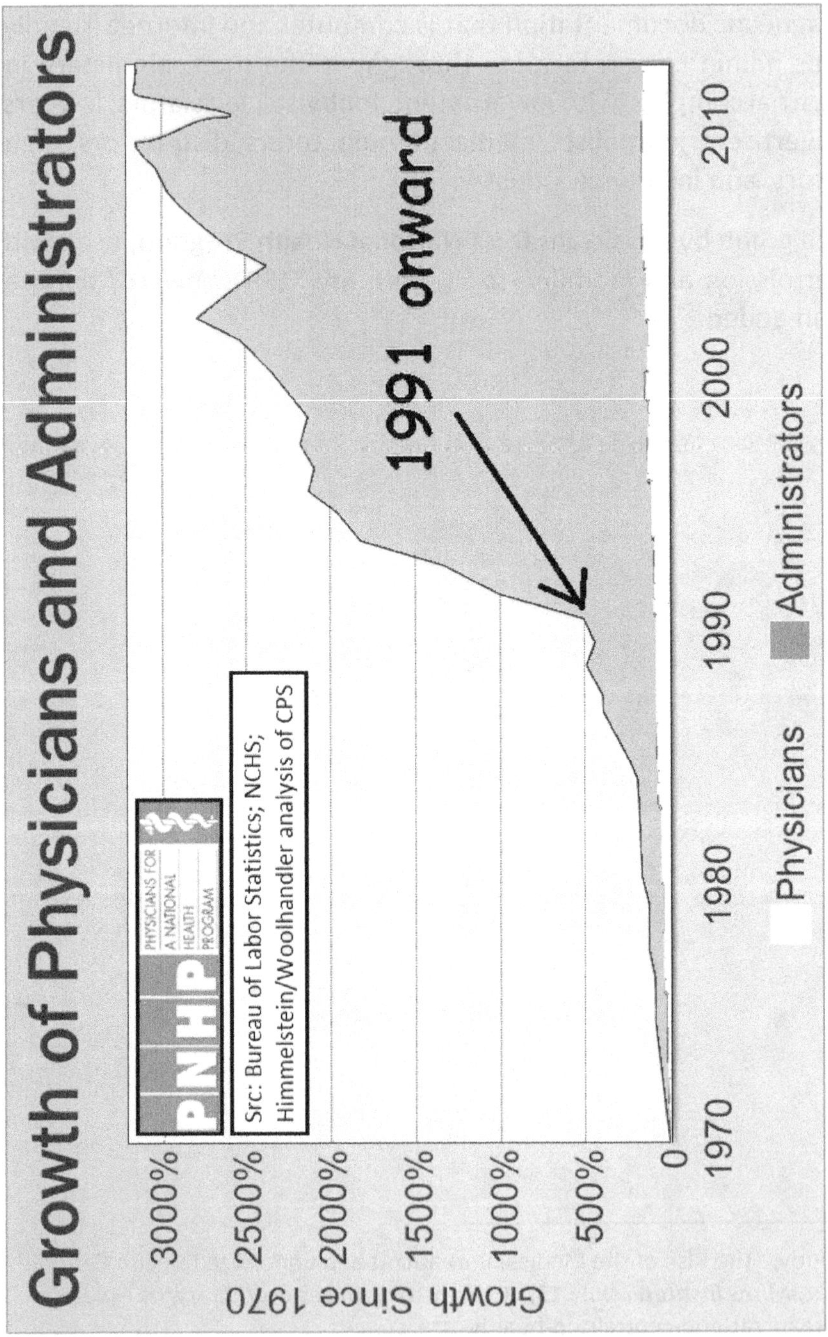
Growth of Physicians and Administrators
Growth Since 1970
3000%
2500%
2000%
1500%
1000%
500%
0
1970
1980
1990
2000
2010
PNHP
PHYSICIANS FOR A NATIONAL HEALTH PROGRAM
Src: Bureau of Labor Statistics; NCHS; Himmelstein/Woolhandler analysis of CPS
1991 onward
Physicians
Administrators

Industrial interest is an apparent root cause of escalating disease, especially in the United States, where compared to other industrial nations, per capita medical cost is the highest while per capita health is among the lowest.

Another timeline correlation is the historical frequency of two words ("ultrasound" and "autism") in books. The following graph is rendered from the Google Ngrams Viewer. Annotations in black are mine. Google limits the upper date range to year 2008.

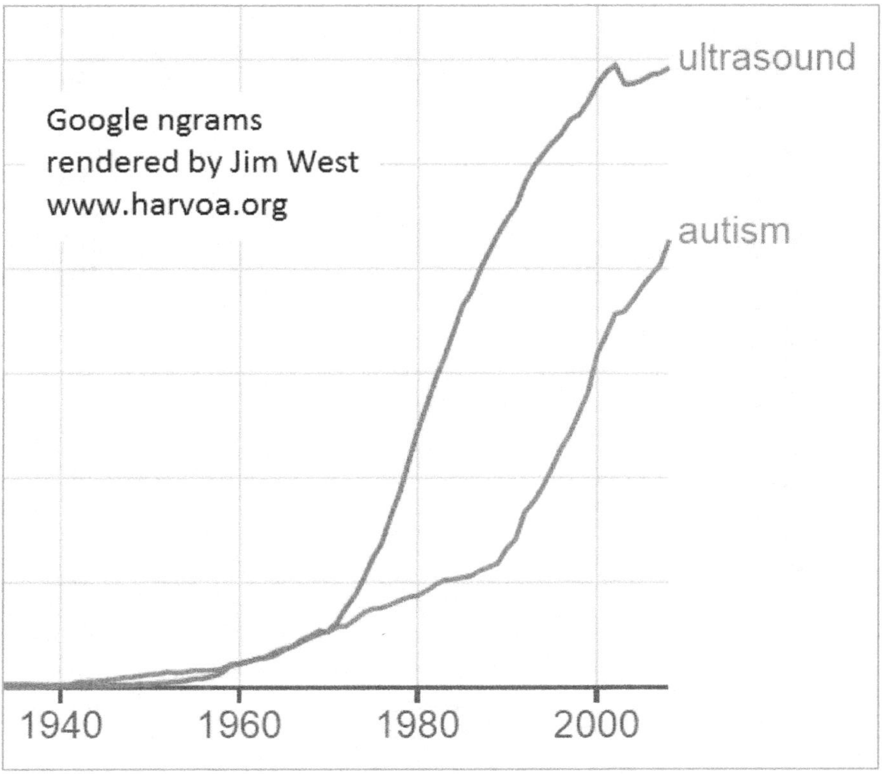

From DUS Book 1, here is the timeline graph of DUS machine intensities (median) versus autism incidence.

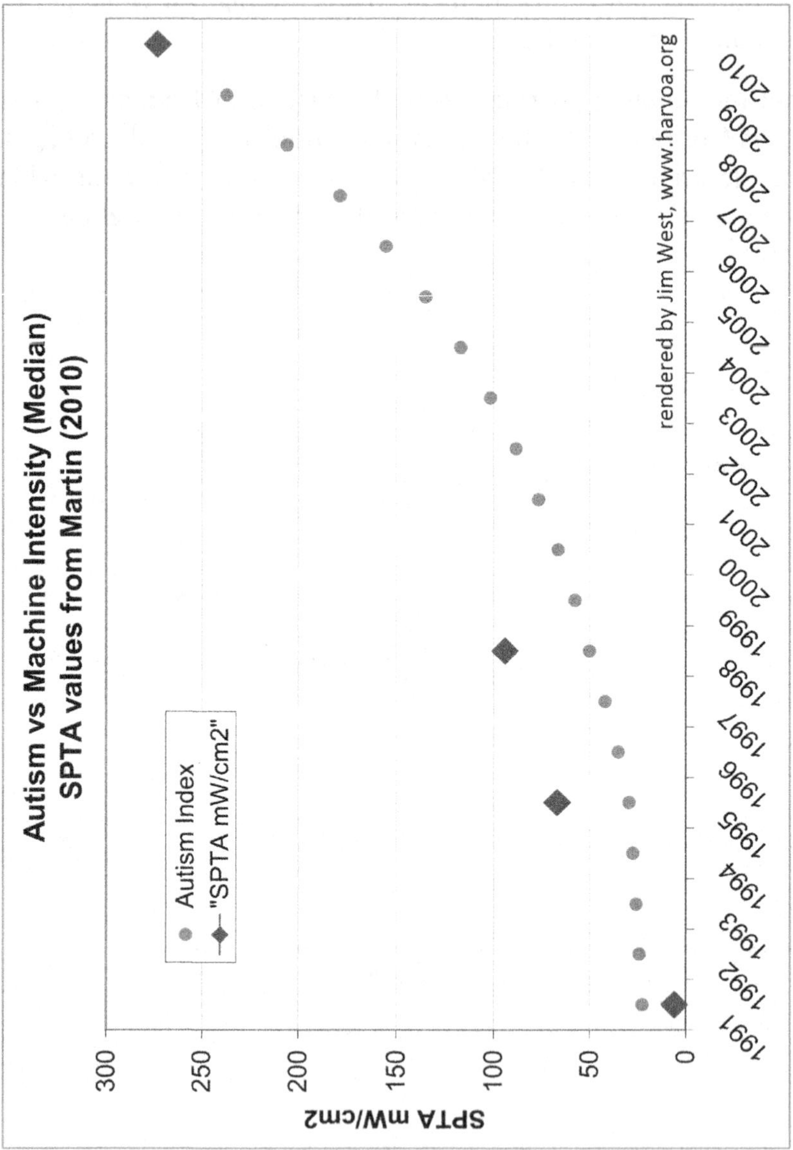

The next graph is a composite of six timelines: newborn weight reduction, rising autism incidence[64], rising DUS intensities[65], rising medical administration class, etc. Note the relation to year 1991, when the FDA increased allowable machine intensities by 8x-15x. All six timelines are indexed at high value = 1.00

[64] AutismSpeaks.org, "Autism Prevalence on the Rise," 2009, https://www.autismspeaks.org/docs/Prevalence_Graph_12_18_2009.pdf.

[65] Kevin Martin, "The Acoustic Safety of New Ultrasound Technologies," Ultrasound 18, no. 3 (August 1, 2010): 110–18, doi:10.1258/ult.2010.010024.

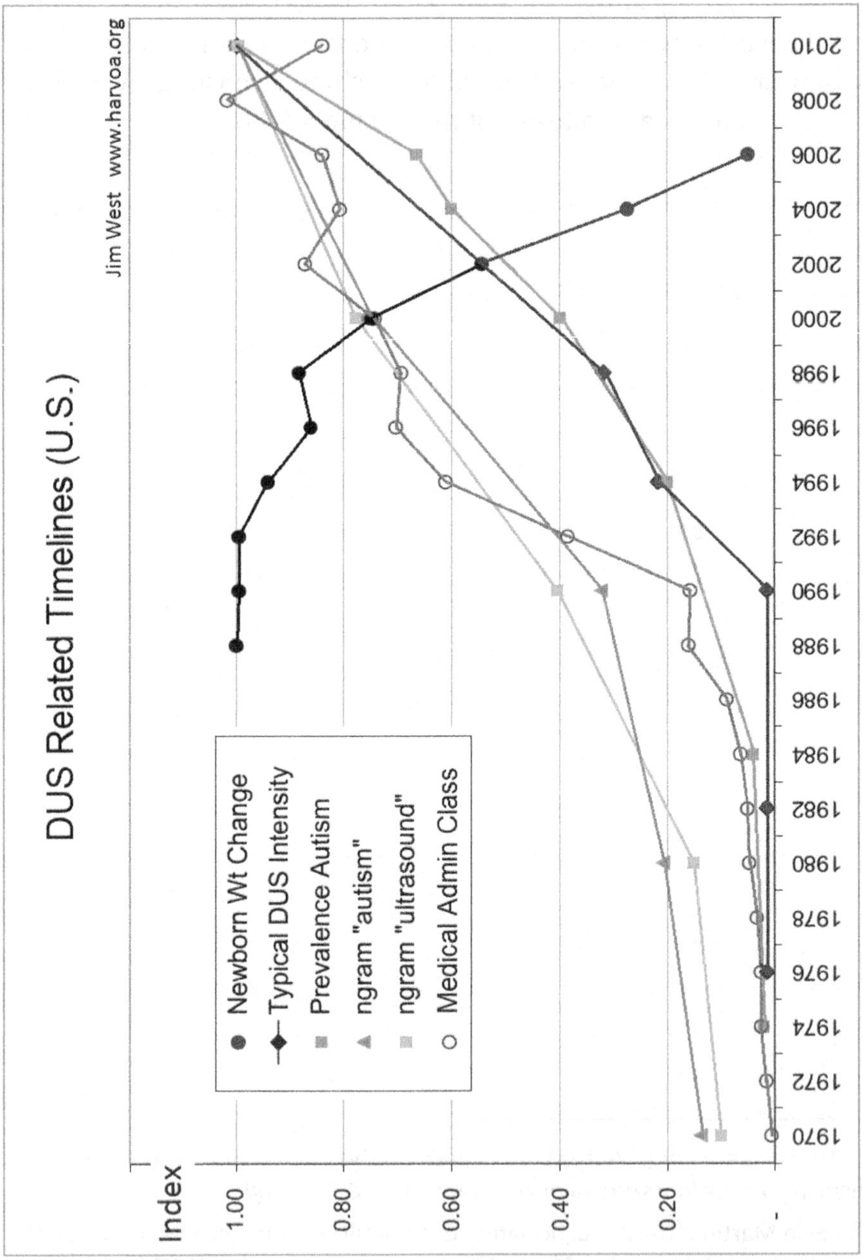
DUS Related Timelines (U.S.)
Jim West www.harvoa.org
Index
1.00
0.80
0.60
0.40
0.20
Newborn Wt Change
Typical DUS Intensity
Prevalence Autism
ngram "autism"
ngram "ultrasound"
Medical Admin Class
1970
1972
1974
1976
1978
1980
1982
1984
1986
1988
1990
1992
1994
1996
1998
2000
2002
2004
2006
2008
2010

Microcephaly Prevalence (U.S. vs Brazil)

CDC declares microcephaly prevalence in the U.S. at 0.07% (7 of 10,000).[66]

Ashwal (2009) calculated that childhood microcephaly prevalence based on normal distribution should be much higher, 2.3% microcephaly for the U.S. population.

> *If Head Circumference is normally distributed, 2.3% of children should by definition be microcephalic. However, published estimates for HC<-2 Standard Deviation at birth are far lower, at 0.56% and 0.54%.*

Ashwal cites reported mild and severe cases, at 0.55% of neonatal population. Severe cases are accurately reported at 0.14% because they are obvious. Mild cases are not reported accurately because they are not obvious. Because most cases are mild, the reported prevalence of 0.55% can be understood as far too low.[67]

Ashwal cites a classroom study of 1,006 students of normal intelligence, finding 1.9% mild microcephaly.

U.S. microcephaly epidemic

Here is another way to estimate U.S. prevalence of microcephaly in the neonatal population, which might be more accurate.

---

[66] Janet D. Cragan, "Baseline Prevalence of Birth Defects Associated with Congenital Zika Virus Infection — Massachusetts, North Carolina, and Atlanta, Georgia, 2013–2014," *MMWR. Morbidity and Mortality Weekly Report* 66 (2017), doi:10.15585/mmwr.mm6608a4.

[67] Ashwal (2009) states that U.S. microcephaly prevalence is statistically imprecise. This is due to the late onset of microcephaly after birth, irregular reporting, and/or irregular distribution of severity.

Within *The Network* epidemic, average neonatal microcephaly incidence was 7% mild cases and 0.2% severe cases, accurately determined by measurement and comparison with prior history in a region that rarely experiences microcephaly. Mild cases ranged up to 15% during the epidemic.

This severe case incidence is similar to annual U.S. incidence, that is, 0.20% vs 0.14% respectively.

Repeating for emphasis: The epidemic incidence in *The Network* is horrific, yet in terms of severe cases its average is comparable to U.S. annual incidence, being only 1.4x the annual U.S. incidence (0.20% / 0.14% = 1.4x).

With both percentages (0.20% and 0.14%) in the same mathematical ballpark, they are reliably subject to the same math that can be applied in order to estimate the prevalence of mild microcephaly within the U.S., as follows:

Within *The Network*, the ratio of severe-to-mild incidence is 35x (7% / 0.2% = 35x).

By applying this accurate 35x ratio to the accurate U.S. severe cases (0.14%), the mild case prevalence can be estimated to be 5% of the U.S. population. This assumes similar environmental stressors, though DUS would be the predominant stressor in both the U.S. and *The Network*. Here it is in a table:

Microcephaly prevalence **U.S. Neonatal Population**	
0.55%	Ashwal (2009)
2.30%	Ashwal (2009) estimated

5.00%	Found by applying Brazil's "35x" to U.S. severe cases

This 5.00% estimate might be a conservative estimate as one classroom study of 1,775 normal students in the U.S. found 0.60% severe microcephaly, according to Ashwal.

U.S. MACROcephaly epidemic

U.S. MACROcephaly is arguably a hidden epidemic, even more so than the microcephaly epidemic.

MACROcephaly prevalence determined by applying Gillberg (2009)		
Percent of U.S. Population		
Given: ASD	2.0%	Zablotsky (2015)[68]
Given: ADHD	11.0%	CDC/ADHD (2017)[69]
Given: MACROcephaly % of ADHD	46%	Gillberg (2002), congenital

---

[68] Benjamin Zablotsky, PhD et al, "Estimated Prevalence of Autism and Other Developmental Disabilities Following Questionnaire Changes in the 2014 National Health Interview Survey," *CDC: National Health Statistics Reports* 87 (November 13, 2015), https://www.cdc.gov/nchs/data/nhsr/nhsr087.pdf.

[69] CDC, "ADHD Data & Statistics," *Centers for Disease Control and Prevention*, September 5, 2017, https://www.cdc.gov/ncbddd/adhd/data.html.

Given: MACROcephaly % of ASD	35%	Gillberg (2002), congenital
Calculated results		
MACROcephaly	5.8%	Gillberg (2002) %'s applied to U.S. population ADHD% and ASD%

Note that the above calculation table does not include a type of MACROcephaly called Proportional MACROcephaly (where head and body are both abnormally large). See Chapter 10 | Proportional MACROcephaly.

Widely imbedded media images appear to normalize MACROcephaly. See for example, the enclosed photo from the CDC "Birth Data" webpage. [70] (Caveat: The child portrayed is not a MACROcephaly case, but the camera angle, focal length and lighting serve to normalize MACROcephaly.)

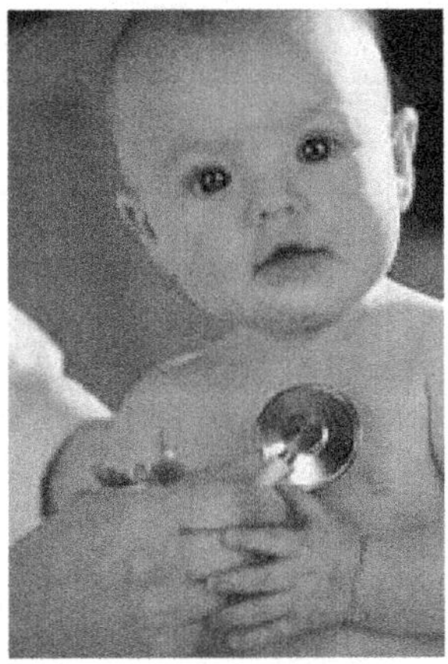

[70] National Vital Statistics System, "Birth Data [CDC]," August 8, 2017, https://www.cdc.gov/nchs/nvss/births.htm.

Assuming there were radiation epidemics in the United States, then where was the public outcry?

The epidemics would have been obfuscated under "congenital rubella", "chorioamnionitis", "infection", "gene mutation", etc.

Isn't this too speculative?

This is reasonable, given the known history of prenatal X-ray carelessness or ruthlessness.

Newnham (1993) population study (DUS)

Newnham is a DUS population study, a case-control study, dose/response study, introduced earlier.

Newnham studied pregnant women attending prenatal clinics May 1989 through November 1991, i.e., during the low intensity era before the great intensity rise (FDA/1991). Newnham's control group received a mere 5mW/cm2 exposure, and its intensive group received also a low intensity Doppler exposure at 25mW/cm2.

Even at these low intensities, Newnham found distinct growth reduction, averaging 25 grams per child. Growth reduction would have been more obvious if the study's low intensity control group were a zero intensity group. With the control group radiated at 5mW/cm2, the results were diluted. Newnham also avoided clarity by not publishing comparisons of DUS session counts vs defect severity.

Newnham still issued a warning:

> *...it would seem prudent to limit ultrasound examinations of the fetus to those cases in which the information is likely to be of clinical importance.*[71]

The warning contains a loophole, "clinical importance", as if any medico would see his use of DUS as not clinically important. Even entertainment DUS ("It's a girl!"), when employed by a medico, is considered clinically important for bonding the mother to her child and bonding the mother to the medico.

O'Brien (1983) mice study (DUS)

William O'Brien, Jr. a prominent researcher at the FDA and the Bioacoustics Research Laboratory. In 1975 and 1976, he conducted a series of mice fetus studies, where he revealed the relation between ultrasound and growth restriction. This study consists of three published papers, 1975, 1976, with a retrospective in 1983.

He used continuous wave ultrasound to radiate 2,865 fetal mice in seven different exposure groups. He found a correlation between growth restriction and ultrasound exposure.

---

[71] J. P. Newnham et al., "Effects of Frequent Ultrasound during Pregnancy: A Randomised Controlled Trial," *Lancet (London, England)* 342, no. 8876 (October 9, 1993): 887–91.

He applied a causation function, relating DUS and growth restriction, dose/response. The function is Intensity^2 x Time. This is represented by O'Brien and the following graph as I^2T.

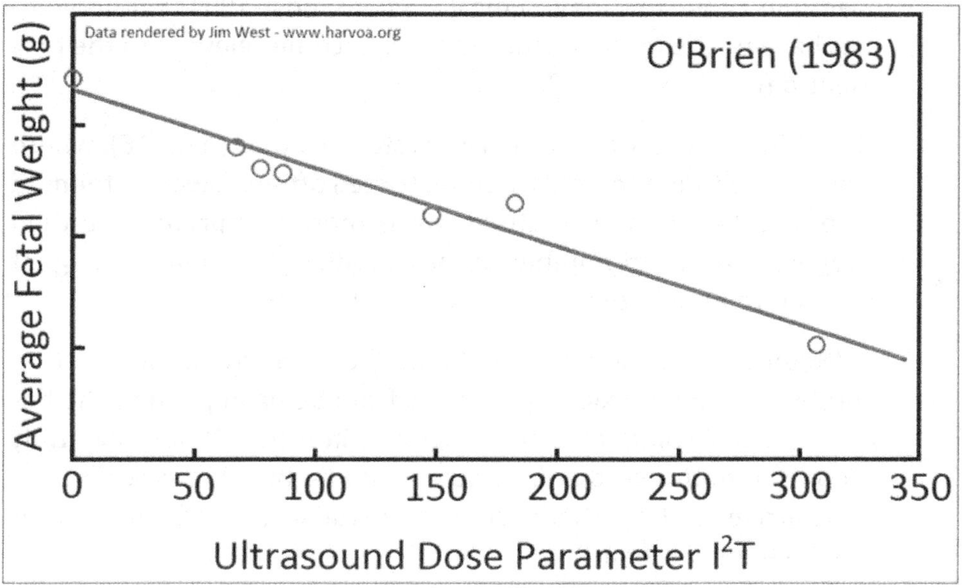

The I^2T function is based on the concept of Dual Radiation Action, described earlier by Kellerer and Rossi (1972).

Relevance

O'Brien studied continuous wave ultrasound on mice fetuses, however, he borrowed the dose/response function, "I^2T" from a prior study of X-ray exposure and carcinogenesis.

He states that the implications of this function would need to be confirmed for clinical settings, because clinical DUS is often pulsed ultrasound, unlike his study of continuous wave ultrasound. He used very high intensity and long dwell times, which puts his exposure levels above the typical clinical scenario circa

1983. Like most published ultrasound studies, his is somewhat inappropriate for clinical relevance, thus ensuring publication.

In 1983, O'Brien may not have anticipated the very high DUS intensities of present-day, clinical sessions, post-1991. Yet his studies have by the mere passage of time become relevant to the present-day.

His study is similar to the Zika virus study by Cugola (2016), where mice were found to be growth-restricted after subjecting them to the so-called Zika virus strain. He is more comprehensive than Cugola in terms of number of mice studied. He studied an agent proven to exist with proven risk, i.e., ultrasound.

O'Brien's caveat nonetheless holds the mainstream dictate that prohibits animal toxicology studies from being applied to the human scenario unless the study benefits industry. That is, his study is only a mouse study not a human study. But that is where the CHS arrive to show that such animal studies are indeed relevant to the human scenario.

Hočevar (2012)

As stated earlier, Hočevar found that low intensity DUS upregulated expression of the Growth Arrest and DNA Damage gene (GADD45a). GADD45a expression is considered a definitive "hallmark" of ionizing radiation (X-rays, etc). Budworth (2012):

> *__DNA damage__ and repair __are hallmarks__ of cellular responses to __ionizing radiation.__*

Ionizing vs Non-Ionizing

Radiation is categorized as "ionizing" and "non-ionizing". Ionizing radiation is more dangerous, examples being extreme ultraviolet light and gamma rays. Ionizing means the capability to dislodge electrons from atoms.

Non-ionizing radiation is declared much safer, incapable of dislodging electrons from atoms. DUS is officially a form of non-ionizing radiation. *Wikipedia* excludes ultrasound from both categories, as if it were not radiation. However, physicists know that ultrasound is a form of non-ionizing radiation. Nevertheless, DUS is usually described as only able to slightly warm tissue, conforming to the ostensible properties of the category, non-ionizing.

Cavitation

Both of those categories fail to describe ultrasound, as ultrasound is capable of triggering atomic fusion and welding steel. Ultrasound can produce cavitational bubbles with core temperatures far higher than the surface of the sun. These are extremely small bubbles. The temperatures are transient, so brief, with a heat energy so quickly absorbed that bioeffects are generally imperceptible, as related bioeffects would occur within the sub-atomic or sub-molecular realms.

To some extent, effects are perceptible, for example, where ultrasound causes fluorescence in water. The nature of this fluorescence is "featureless", somewhat beyond the ability of technical analysis, possibly akin to cyclotron radiation.[72]

If anything could appear harmless, yet destroy that nearest the soul, it would be ultrasound. Those transient but extreme temperatures must be burning something within the nano- or pico-realm in addition to the known grosser damage.

The marketing of DUS is safeguarded by declaring it "harmless", by declaring that "ultrasound is not ionizing radiation like X-rays".

---

[72] Kenneth S. Suslick and David J. Flannigan, "Inside a Collapsing Bubble: Sonoluminescence and the Conditions During Cavitation," *Annual Review of Physical Chemistry* 59 (2008): 659–83.

Hočevar (2012) bridged the two categories (ionizing vs non-ionizing) with his discovery that clinical DUS can increase the expression of GADD45a by a factor far beyond that observed in similar X-ray studies.

7 | Radiation Syndrome

Causation patterns

An original concept of "medical radiation syndrome" is developed that includes DUS. This is necessary because the term is missing from literature.

First, three similar terms are introduced (syndrome, comorbidity, risk factors).

THREE TERMS

Syndrome

A collection of diseases, disorders, conditions, or symptoms, only one of which is necessary for the syndrome name. (Example: Microcephaly syndrome consists of small brain, often with eye, hearing, heart damage, ASD, etc.)

Comorbidity

The co-occurrence of diseases in the same organism. (Example: Microcephaly is often comorbid with eye damage.)

Risk factors

This is a big topic by itself. The term "risk factors" is used three different ways.

1. The diagnosis of disorder A indicates the probable additional diagnosis of disorder B. (Example: Microcephaly is a [diagnostic] risk factor for ASD, eye and hearing damage.)
2. Disorder A can cause disorder B. (Example: IUGR is a [causative] risk factor for autism.)
3. Poison A can cause disorder A. (Example: DUS is a [causative] risk factor for myelination dysfunction. Myelin is a nerve sheath. Myelination is the early growth process whereby myelin forms.)

Usage (of "risk factors')

Everyone uses definition 1.

Toxicologists tend to use definitions 1 and 3.

Clinicians often use definition 2, which fear mongers while avoiding rigorous proof and toxicology. This sells medical intervention by promoting the idea of treating one symptom in order to repress another.

Four examples of "risk factor" use

1) Viruses are declared a causative **risk factor** for cancer.[73] For example, oncologists Nichols and Barrett casually conflate the germ/environment dichotomy as they declare viruses causative

---

[73] "Viruses That Can Lead to Cancer," accessed August 4, 2017, https://www.cancer.org/cancer/cancer-causes/infectious-agents/infections-that-can-lead-to-cancer/viruses.html.

for cancer by association of the two observations (viruses and cancer):

> *Viruses are a risk factor for cancer second only to tobacco.*[74]

2) Intraocular fluid pressure is declared a causative **risk factor** for glaucoma, rationalizing toxic drug treatments (e.g., Brimonidine) to lower pressure. Causative evidence is speculative "despite intense efforts" to prove causation by ocular pressure.[75] This approach is a hazard because toxic drug treatments would compound the toxicity of what may already be an environmental disease. Pharmaceuticals give false impressions of improvement due to their hormesis effects, thereby diffusing any efforts to determine causation.

3) Fever is declared a causative **risk factor** for brain damage, with drugs then prescribed to lower fever. Yet fever is also known to be a natural response to poisoning. Toxic drugs like Tylenol or aspirin are prescribed to "fight" the fever, yet, these would compound any prior toxicity that may have initiated the fever response.

4) Autism literature contains language such as the following, from, *Autism Spectrum Disorders,* by Amaral (2011).[76]

---

[74] "Research Projects in the Mymryk Laboratory," accessed August 4, 2017, http://publish.uwo.ca/~jmymryk/projects.html.

[75] John Berdahl, MD, "Cerebrospinal Fluid Pressure and Glaucoma," *Glaucoma Today*, October 2009, 14.

[76] David Amaral, Geraldine Dawson, and Daniel Geschwind, *Autism Spectrum Disorders* (Oxford University Press, USA, 2011), 1265.

> *...risk factors contribute to risk processes resulting in secondary effects of the early symptoms that may contribute to the development of the full ASD syndrome...*

This is another example of risk factors implying mutual causation. Such inward pointing theories generate fear and avenues for exploitive treatments while avoiding toxicology.

Amaral (2011) advocates intervention:

> *By intervening early before the full syndrome is present, it might be possible to mitigate the downstream effects of early symptoms on later...*

Advocates toxic drugs:

> *...combined pharmacological and behavioral approach...*

Advocates funding:

> *Research reflecting the reality of providing multimodal interventions will have the largest impact in the care of individuals with autism. Such studies are fairly difficult to do and require significant commitment on the part of funding agencies...*

DUS Syndrome

A microcephaly-related concept of "DUS Syndrome" will now be developed.

Congenital microcephaly is comorbid with many diseases. Hollander (2000):

> *In 25 out of 30 infants [with microcephaly], microcephaly proved to be part of a complex problem.*[77]

Zika virus syndrome (CVS) is similar to congenital rubella syndrome (CRS), and both are common to microcephaly syndrome.

> *"What we learned about rubella and pregnancy, and how we learned it — we are definitely looking to those lessons as we learn more every day about Zika virus," said Peggy Honein [CDC].*[78]

Congenital Rubella Syndrome

Congenital Zika virus syndrome and congenital rubella virus syndrome are similar. Common symptoms are microcephaly, IUGR, eye, hearing, heart disorders, ASD, ADHD, developmental delays, skin rash, etc. (Details in Part B).

In 1941, CRS was discovered.[79] This was during the era of careless prenatal X-ray exposure. Though discovered, CRS had a long but un-named prior epidemic history.

---

[77] NS Den Hollander et al., "Congenital Microcephaly Detected by Prenatal Ultrasound: Genetic Aspects and Clinical Significance," *Ultrasound in Obstetrics and Gynecology* 15, no. 4 (April 1, 2000): 282–87, doi:10.1046/j.1469-0705.2000.00092.x.

[78] Adrienne LaFrance, "What Zika Researchers Can Learn From the Rubella Outbreak of 1964," *The Atlantic*, April 6, 2016, https://www.theatlantic.com/health/archive/2016/04/zika-rubella/477165/.

[79] CDC, "Rubella | Epidemiology of Vaccine Preventable Diseases," accessed August 3, 2017, https://www.cdc.gov/vaccines/pubs/pinkbook/rubella.html#rubella.

In contrast, CZS, the Brazil epidemic, is described by the mainstream as originating unprecedented, in Brazil, during 2015. However, CZS apparently also had a long epidemic history in the U.S. and in other more developed nations.

Note that CRS dominates diagnoses wherever it competes with suspected X-ray damage. Stevenson (2005):

> *Any attempt to study the prevalence of microcephaly is* ***challenged by a discouraging array*** *of methodologic problems... The causal mix of microcephaly should show a... change as certain causes are largely* ***eliminated (congenital rubella)****...*[80]

Thus...

Before the late 1970s, rubella syndrome would better be named "X-ray syndrome.[81]

After the late 1970s, when "harmless" DUS began replacing prenatal X-ray sessions, "DUS Syndrome" would be the better name.

Medicos already use the unsupported term "Zika virus syndrome", so why not the well-supported term, "DUS Syndrome"?

Medicos would object: "We don't diagnose a disease already knowing the cause. We observe the symptoms then deduce the cause."

Their hypocrisy is evident with their long tradition of presuming infection without evidence. Proof? The reader need only recall his

---

[80] Roger E. Stevenson, Dir and Judith G. Hall Professor of Pediatrics University of British Columbia, *Human Malformations and Related Anomalies* (Oxford University Press, USA, 2005), 498.

[81] The term, "X-ray syndrome", is apparently unprecedented. "Radiation sickness" exists; "acute radiation syndrome" exists, however, not "X-ray syndrome".

own experience with medicos routinely declaring infection without evidence, while prescribing toxic antibiotics and sedatives.

In terms of microcephaly causation, the known X-ray science, when compared to the available DUS science, assists in the discovery of the Zika virus cover story. This discovery in turn reveals its predecessor, the rubella virus cover story (for X-ray damage).

CRS is a major disinfo germ paradigm for prenatal X-ray damage. The great congenital rubella epidemics of the 20th century were caused by prenatal X-rays.

It is incredible but true that generally, when medicos declare infection causative for neonatal disease, symptoms are deemed conclusive evidence for infection even when actual germs are not found. Mere fever is enough for a diagnosis of prenatal infection (thereby avoiding toxicology). For example, see the chorioamnionitis paradigm finely deconstructed in Part B.

Maternal rubella (non-congenital)

The official definition for non-congenital rubella (child, adult, or maternal) is, "a viral disease like measles", "3-day measles", "German measles", and "maternal rubella".

The non-congenital version is different from the congenital version (CRS). It is known by its measles-like rash. It is mild, while CRS is devastating. All versions are declared causative by the rubella virus. The worldwide epidemics of 1963-1965 are explored in Part B.

The benefits of deceit

Fake rubella and Zika virus paradigms are useful. They protect industry of course. They allow coded discussions of sensitive issues, thereby stabilizing technocracy. Even the individual can benefit from virus paradigms.

A positive test result for a "virus" can serve as a useful toxicological warning to expectant mothers, for it has long been known that increases in the amount of nucleic acid fragments are "toxicity biomarkers". And, viruses have long been officially defined as "rogue nucleic acid".[82] "Nucleic acid fragments" and "rogue nucleic acid" must be the same thing if the reader can dismiss the concept of a predatory virus, and he certainly can (see prior topic "Virus Causation").

Maternal rubella syndrome (rashes, blisters, redness, fever, inflammation, etc.) should be viewed as evidence of X-ray or DUS damage in the fetal region. The non-maternal child-adult rubella version should be viewed in terms of other forms of pollution, such as pesticide pollution, before entertaining germ theories.

Though maternal rubella is comparatively harmless to the mother, the related fetal damage, when later presenting severely in the newborn, is commonly misdiagnosed as an infection (CRS, chorioamnionitis, Group B Strep (GBS), Zika virus, etc.) The danger is real fetal damage from DUS, and the diagnostic alarm bells can bring hazardous intervention cascades. Once the scenario is created, the mother has few good options.

If a pregnant woman is diagnosed with maternal rubella syndrome (diagnosed by symptoms), there is a 85% that her newborn will have CRS, as indicated by Dawe (2007):

> *About 85% of fetuses with mothers who become infected [with rubella virus] before the 20th week will develop CRS [Congenital Rubella Syndrome].*[83]

---

[82] Respectively, the work of Howard Urnovitz, PhD, and, *Encyclopedia Britannica Micropaedia*, "virus".

[83] Halley Dawe, "Rubella" (Microbiology Department, Austin Community College, 2007), http://www.austincc.edu/microbio/2704r/rv.htm.

A medico should consider that the stated maternal rubella syndrome is actually DUS Syndrome. Just replace virus terms with radiation terms, as follows:

> *About 85% of fetuses of mothers who present an inflammatory response (fever and rash) to medical radiation before the 20th week gestation, will develop congenital radiation syndrome.*[84]

Then investigate the woman's radiation history. If nothing is found then the medico can always return to the infectious paradigm.

The formula

During the present era of prenatal DUS exposure, Zika virus is a cover story for both neonatal and maternal DUS damage.

Congenital Zika Syndrome (CZS) (as DUS damage) is similar to Congenital Rubella Syndrome (CRS) (as X-ray damage).

Consider this reflection in Rasmussen (2016):

> *...if **Zika virus** is similar to other teratogens, an expansion of the phenotype would be expected, for example, **with the congenital rubella syndrome...***

Note that during the Brazil "Zika" epidemic, officials had a big problem differentiating CRS from CZS. Early studies of the epidemic actually reported finding rubella "virus" antibodies in nearly all microcephaly cases. (Details in Part C.)

---

[84] Dawe (2007) rewritten by Jim West in terms of medical radiation, for a contrasting view

SYNDROME

Any syndrome or spectrum can be re-ordered as in the matrix below to show its comorbid disorders, and all point to one presumed initiating cause, DUS.

Congenital Disease Syndromes			
Microcephaly Syndrome	**Growth Restriction Syndrome**	**MACRO-cephaly Syndrome**	**Autism Spectrum Disorder**
•	Microcephaly Syndrome	Microcephaly Syndrome	Microcephaly Syndrome
Growth Restriction Syndrome	•	Growth Restriction Syndrome	Growth Restriction Syndrome
MACRO-cephaly Syndrome	MACRO-cephaly Syndrome	•	MACRO-cephaly Syndrome
Autism Spectrum Disorder	Autism Spectrum Disorder	Autism Spectrum Disorder	•
etc.	etc.	etc.	etc.

MICROCEPHALY SYNDROME

Reconsider the syndrome matrix as a spoked wheel.

Microcephaly syndrome usually consists of many possible disorders, which can be portrayed as a syndrome wheel.

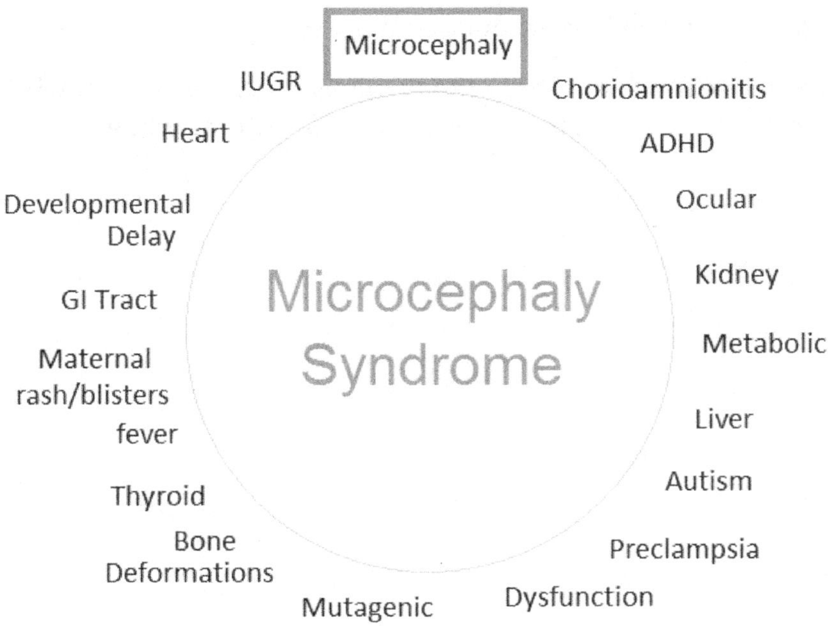

IUGR SYNDROME

IUGR ("intrauterine growth restriction") is like microcephaly but determined by abdomen size rather than head size. Some call it a spectrum rather than a syndrome because it can include syndromes.[85]

---

[85] Francesc Figueras, MD and Jason Gardosi, MD, FRCOG, "Intrauterine Growth Restriction: New Concepts in Antenatal Surveillance, Diagnosis, and

Muia (2014) declares that IUGR is a leading ***"cause"*** of infant mortality:

> *...Nearly half of all infant mortality occurs in the first 28 days after birth with Intrauterine Growth Restriction (IUGR) syndrome being one of the* ***leading causes****...*[86]

Of course, it should be argued that IUGR is just one of many biological responses to environmental stress.

See the next wheel, where the previous Autism Spectrum wheel is rotated one notch to display an IUGR Syndrome wheel.

Management," *AJOG*, August 7, 2010, http://www.gestation.net/PDFs/IUGR_new_concepts_AJOG_Review.pdf.

[86] Caroline Muia, Chunyu Lu, and Ajoy Basak, "An Efficient and Selective in Vitro Solid Phase Assay for PCSK4 Activity: Potential Diagnostic Tool in Fetal and Placental Growth Restriction," April 15, 2014, https://www.ruor.uottawa.ca/bitstream/10393/30871/1/Muia_Caroline.pdf.

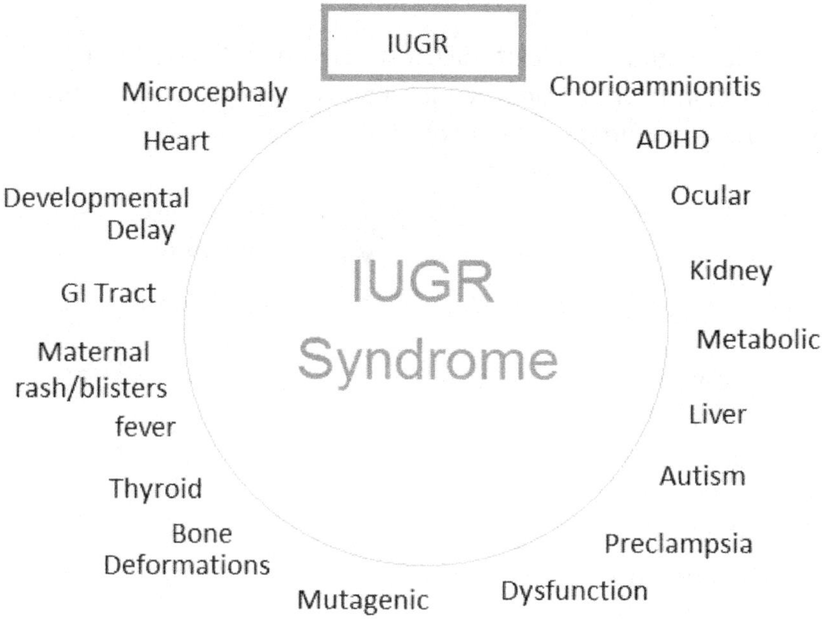
IUGR
IUGR Syndrome
Microcephaly
Heart
Developmental Delay
GI Tract
Maternal rash/blisters fever
Thyroid
Bone Deformations
Mutagenic
Chorioamnionitis
ADHD
Ocular
Kidney
Metabolic
Liver
Autism
Preclampsia
Dysfunction

ASD (Spectrum)

Autism is the main topic of ASD, a spectrum (collection of possible disorders and syndromes), which can be represented by turning the aforesaid wheel a few notches.

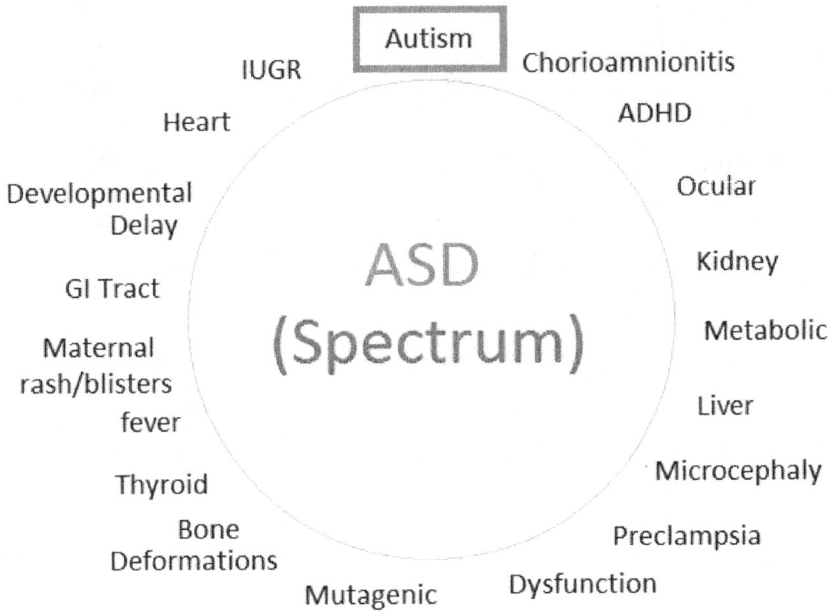

DUS Syndrome

The DUS Syndrome wheel is pragmatic simplicity. Rotation not required. The most obvious disease would be highlighted per discussion, reflecting the diverse reality of the NE Brazil epi-

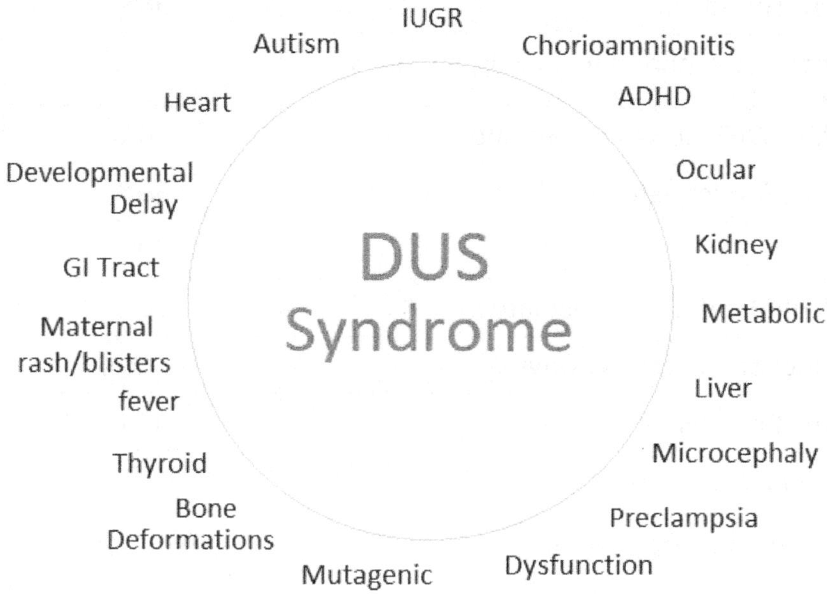

demic.

Context

Though DUS Syndrome is arguably the dominant cause of child disease, there are other environmental contributors. Stepping back for context, the following table presents my rough estimate of fetal stressor exposure.

Prominence of Fetal Stressors Listed as My INVERSION of the Mainstream View	Stress to the Fetal Population as Index: 0-100%
Ultrasound	98%
Antibiotics, pharmaceuticals, vaccines	45%
EMF: WiFi, power cables and devices[87]	30%
Stove/Boiler exhaust	30%
X-rays	20%
Alcohol/caffeine/chocolate	30%
Infection - bacteria/fungus	2%
Infection - virus	0%

*Alcohol is a teratogen.

Dr. Svetlana Popova warns:

> *There is no safe amount of alcohol, no safe time and no safe type of alcohol to drink during pregnancy... completely avoid alcohol for at least two months before conception.*[88]

---

[87] "Electric blankets increase risk of miscarriage: study - Korea Biomedical Review," January 2, 2018, http://www.koreabiomed.com/news/articleView.html?idxno=2179.

[88] Claire Gagne, "A New Study on Drinking During Pregnancy Draws Alarming Conclusions," *Today's Parent*, January 7, 2016, http://www.todaysparent.com/pregnancy/being-pregnant/a-new-study-on-drinking-during-pregnancy-draws-alarming-conclusions/.

Alcoholism could be a symptom of other risk factors not discounted, e.g., carelessness, ignorance, gullibility, and passive victimhood, signaling a free-for-all.

8 | Tip of the Iceberg

View from the Titanic

The most obvious disease is merely the epidemic name. Dr. Albert Ko (2016) finds more to the microcephaly epidemic:

> *...microcephaly may just be the tip of the iceberg... [some] babies who don't have microcephaly may also have neurological lesions or birth defects that are not as obvious as microcephaly.*[89]

This diverse syndrome does not require microcephaly. Costello (2016):

> *... babies [**with normal head circumference, without microcephaly**] have been reported to have **neurological** abnor-*

---

[89] "Zika Expert: 'Microcephaly May Just Be the Tip of the Iceberg.,'" *Washington Post*, accessed September 16, 2016, https://www.washingtonpost.com/news/to-your-health/wp/2016/02/09/zika-expert-microcephaly-may-just-be-the-tip-of-the-iceberg/.

> *malities... the **genital, urinary, cardiac** and **digestive** systems can be affected (Pilar Ramon-Pardo, unpublished data).*[90]

Distribution curve

See graphic distribution of the diverse epidemic.

Using known and estimated data, the non-diagnosed and non-diagnosable diseases can be estimated re the epidemic of NE Brazil. Future reports should confirm what is already being observed by clinicians such as Dr. Ko, and eventually, years later, confirm childhood and adult diseases.

The highest estimates (not shown) would represent the non-diagnosable diseases, such as damage to the spark of life, courage, personality, sensitivity, and common profundity.

The extent of damage would depend on the complex variances of DUS exposure and bad luck, i.e., operator experience, safety knowledge and habits, dwell-time, intensity, number of sessions, length of sessions, hardware compliance, etc.

---

[90] Anthony Costello et al., "Defining the Syndrome Associated with Congenital Zika Virus Infection," *Bulletin of the World Health Organization* 94, no. 6 (June 1, 2016): 406–406A, doi:10.2471/BLT.16.176990.

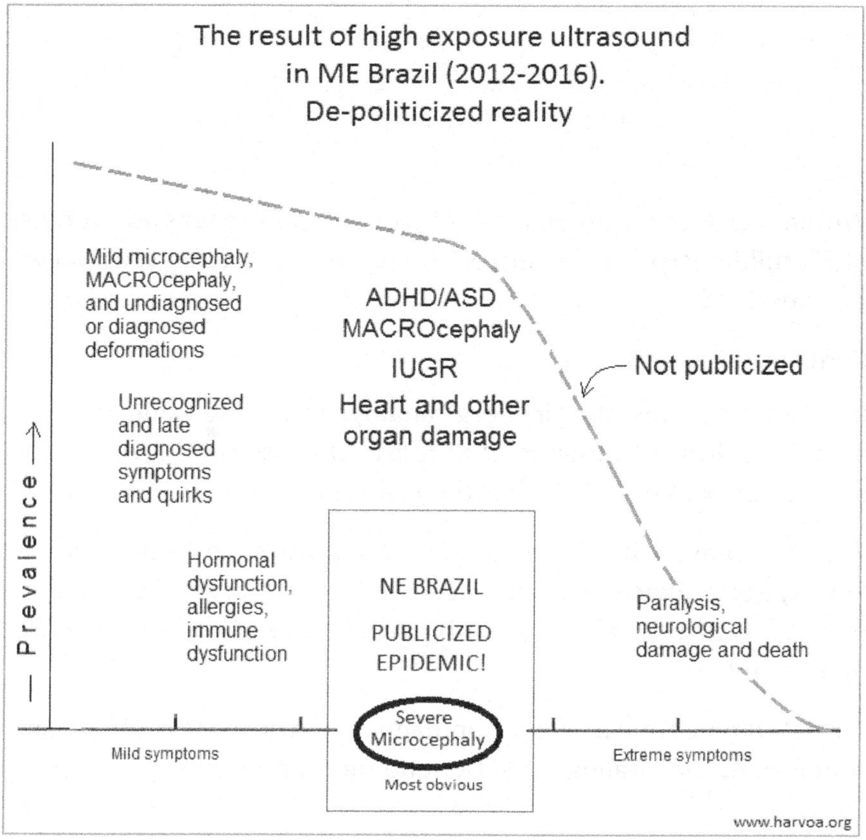

Erin's 100%

Erin, a mother conversing on Chris Kessler's online forum, supports this view of omnipresent pathology. She sees the extended prevalence of ASD in 100% of those with multiple DUS sessions:

> *Would a slightly weakened immune system be apparent at birth? Or some mild-severe neurological problems? There are so many crazy new disorders and diseases with babies these days... Personally, 100% of the babies of friends I've had who had multiple ultrasounds have had issues with*

> *sleeping as babies, and having worse than normal immune systems, babies that get sick ALL the time. And as toddlers they seem slightly autistic or "off" socially... not enough for them to be considered autistic, but enough to see when all the kids get together, which ones are "different".*[91]

Within the birth population of *The Network*, there was an average of 7% mild microcephaly and 0.2% severe microcephaly, as of December 2015.

Conceptual stretch

If we were to apply the "iceberg" analogy to the 7% value, we find a DUS Syndrome epidemic of at least 70% (an iceberg tip represents approximately 1/10th of the iceberg).

70% is a reasonable ballpark value because even in the United States, neurological disorders for children are diagnosed at 15% (i.e., 11% with ADHD,[92] 2.2% with ASD,[93] and 2% other developmental delay[94]).

A related epidemic of milder undiagnosed disorders could be another 15%, subtotaling 30%. Depending on how subtly filtered is

---

[91] "Natural Childbirth IIb: Ultrasound Not as Safe as Commonly Thought [10/6/2016]," *Chris Kresser*, July 15, 2011, https://chriskresser.com/natural-childbirth-iib-ultrasound-not-as-safe-as-commonly-thought/.

[92] J. Fayyad et al., "Cross-National Prevalence and Correlates of Adult Attention-Deficit Hyperactivity Disorder," *The British Journal of Psychiatry* 190, no. 5 (May 1, 2007): 402–9, doi:10.1192/bjp.bp.106.034389.

[93] Benjamin Zablotsky, PhD et al, "Estimated Prevalence of Autism and Other Developmental Disabilities Following Questionnaire Changes in the 2014 National Health Interview Survey."

[94] CDC, NCBDDD, "Developmental Disabilities," accessed August 3, 2017, https://www.cdc.gov/ncbddd/developmentaldisabilities/about.html.

the rest of the distribution curve, and including hormetic opposites, such as MACROcephaly, this could be more than 70% of the population, to some degree, and in view of the CHS etc., approximating Erin's 100%.

Ed Arranga of *AutismOne* posts a similar view and backs it up with statistics:

> *A staggering 54% percent of American children are chronically ill. One child in 68 has autism, and attention-deficit/hyperactivity disorder affects approximately 11% of the country's children. At least 1 child in 6 has a developmental disorder. The special education system is buckling beneath the weight of 13% of American children using special education.*[95]

Ed then pushes the vaccine causation paradigm. I received no reply to my attempts to alert AutismOne of the primacy of DUS hazards.

---

[95] Ed Arranga, "'The Cost of Autism' Web App to Be Unveiled by AutismOne Explores the Economic Cost of Vaccine Injury to the Nation," *Cision: PRweb*, October 27, 2017, http://www.prweb.com/releases/2017/10/prweb14853256.htm.

9 | Hormesis

Truer dose/response curves

Scientific perception of toxicity requires some sense of a dose/response relationship, yet this is often deficient in DUS causation science. Consider the word "hormesis", for example.

Riviere (2006), a standard toxicology textbook, describes a monumental "error":

> *[During the] mid-20th century... the toxicology community made an error...* **concerning the nature of dose-response***. During this crucial period of... toxicological intellectual imprinting... the threshold dose/response model became accepted while* **the hormesis model... became fully marginalized.** *The hormetic dose/response model that had developed a reasonably large database,* **was not to be included** *in the major textbooks on toxicology and pharmacology, was omitted from academic courses... was excluded*

> *from... regulatory agencies. This... continuing to the present... represents **a clear form of intellectual censorship**.*[96]

Accents the profundity of this "censorship":

> *...the toxicological community [rejected] **the hormetic dose/response model.... the most fundamental principle and pillar of toxicology**... enormous implications for how toxicology is conducted, how its studies are designed, how risks are assessed...*

The "error" made real science virtually illegal. In his autobiography, *Truth in a Life of Science*, the toxicologist, Andrew A. Marino, PhD, describes his creative handling of similar NIH (National Institutes of Health) repression.[97]

Studies often ignore and play games with hormesis. They average out results from different parts of the hormesis response curve without admitting that hormesis exists. They interpret results as irrational by pretending to be unaware of hormesis. The censorship and corruption of the word "hormesis" is comparable to the assignment of AAA ratings to Junk Bonds prior to the 2008 Bubble Crash.

Science authors often present somewhat truthful data then conclude falsely according to the prevailing censorship required to gain publication. Yet in their studies, politically sensitive data is still available to the discerning reader.

---

[96] Jim E. Riviere, *Biological Concepts and Techniques in Toxicology: An Integrated Approach* (CRC Press, 2006), 86.

[97] Andrew Marino, PhD, *Going Somewhere: Truth About a Life in Science* (Cassandra Publishing, 2011).

The usual (hormesis not considered)

People tend to see toxicity related to inhibitory and dysfunctional responses, i.e., the more poison, the more dysfunction.

Mathematically this would be seen as a downward linear dose/ response, e.g., Toxicity x Time = Dysfunction, pain and suffering. This is somewhat valid, but it does not accurately describe toxicity, especially mild toxicity, which is omnipresent in industrial society. See next graph.

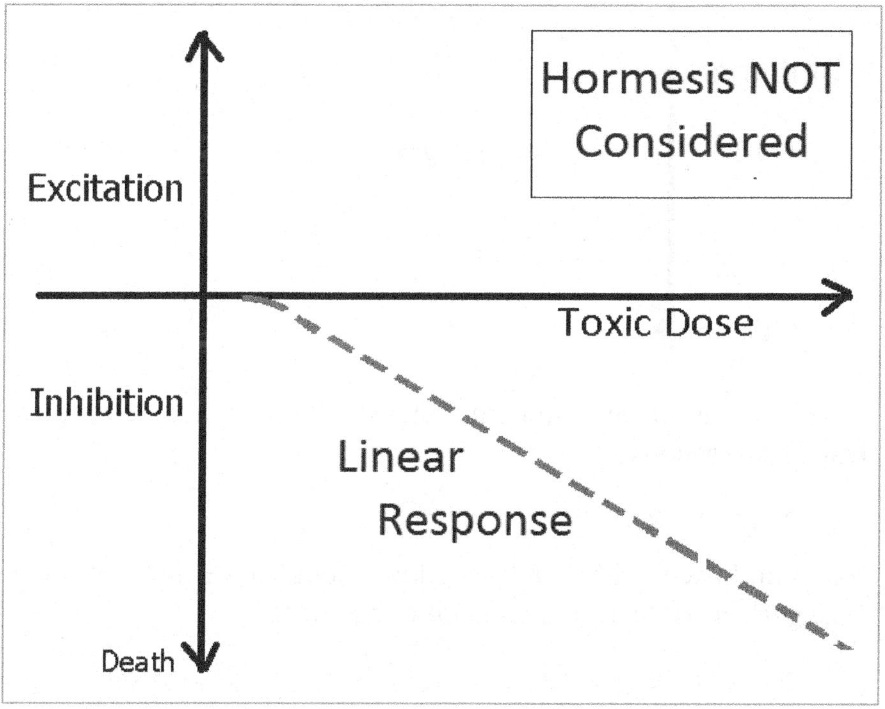

A similar dose/response curve, often used by scientists, is the "S-Curve". This is similar to the pure linear response curve above in that all responses are negative for any toxic dose. See next graph.

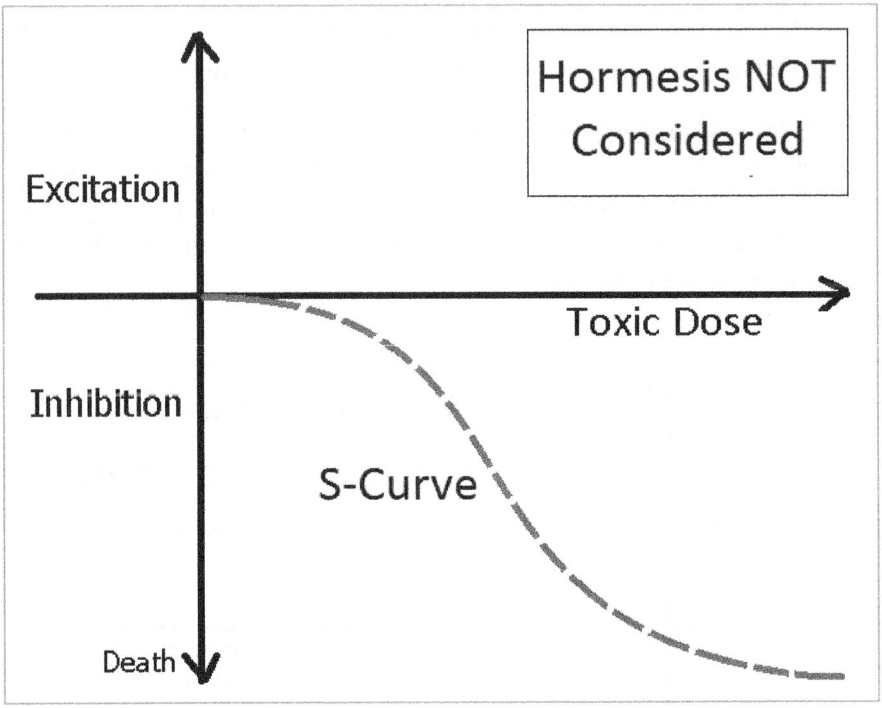

The S-curve is an improvement, but it still does not accurately portray dose/response.

Hormesis explored

Hayes and Laws (1991), in its section, "Beneficial Effects Of Small Dosages", introduces the concept of hormesis:

> *...bacteriologist Hueppe (1896) stated the rule... "Every substance that kills and destroys protoplasm in certain concentrations inhibits development in lower concentrations, but acts as a stimulus and increases the potential of*

life at even lower concentrations beyond a point of neutrality.[98]

Hormesis is sensible

When life is obviously poisoned, it tries to evade the poisoning by abatement, catharsis and distance. When mildly poisoned, an organism may not know it is poisoned, but its cellular and hormonal systems respond by accelerating metabolism. This rise in activity increases survival options. The organism, still unaware, may feel unusually happy and optimistic, but simultaneously, vulnerabilities increase, such as bad judgment.

This is typically represented by a hormesis bump at the beginning of a dose/response curve. See graph.

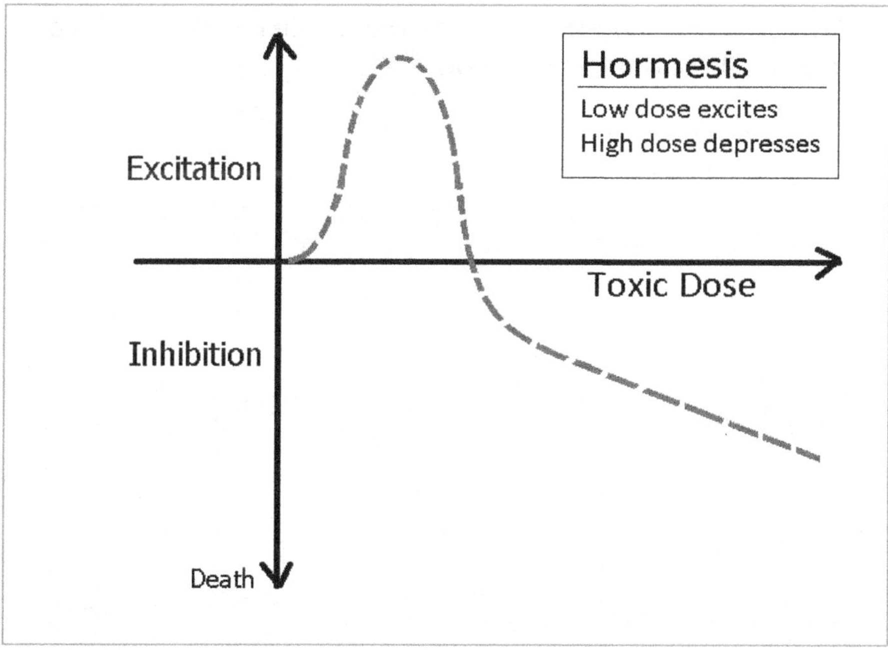

[98] Wayland J. Hayes and Edward R. Laws, *Handbook of Pesticide Toxicology: General Principles* (Academic Press, 1991), 59.

Industrial spin

Modern Medicine interprets hormesis to its advantage. When it cannot ignore this word, it mischaracterizes it by defining hormetic symptoms on the left side of the curve (the bump) as "beneficial".

Social strategists use the hormesis concept to ennoble mass poisoning as a necessary social challenge. Hayes and Laws (1991):

> *The term "sufficient challenge"... emphasizes the need of the organism for some measure of stress... a small amount of poison... Toynbee's concept of "sufficient but not overpowering challenge" in connection with human history.*[99]

With the word, "hormesis", *Wikipedia* is able to describe the effects of mild poisoning as "favorable":

> *Hormesis is the term for generally **favorable** biological responses to low exposures to toxins and other stressors... A pollutant or toxin showing hormesis thus has the opposite effect in small doses as in large doses.*[100]

---

[99] Jim West, "Rationale for Industrial Poisoning," *Images of Poliomyelitis*, 2001, http://harpub.tk/toxcredo.htm.

[100] "Hormesis," *Wikipedia*, May 8, 2016, https://en.wikipedia.org/w/index.php?title=Hormesis&oldid=719252509.

Mattson (2008) promotes toxic pharmaceuticals with "hormesis":

> *A better understanding of hormesis mechanisms at the cellular and molecular levels is leading to novel approaches [pharmaceuticals] for the prevention and treatment of many different diseases.*[101]

Promotes the dubious concept of immunization to poisoning, by employing the hormesis concept:

> *...an organism might benefit by having its immune system stimulated by low doses of a contaminant, so that it is 'prepared' for higher doses.*

The viability of such a pollution vaccine is debatable. Such vaccines would complicate the environmental diagnostic picture, thereby undermining toxicology. Such vaccines would attack the vulnerable.

Robert McNamara (deceased, former President of The World Bank, U.S. Secretary of State, etc.) omits hormesis as he promotes a sensationalist view of population control:

> *One must take draconian measures... against the will of the populations. Reducing the birth rate has proved to be impossible or insufficient. One must therefore increase the mortality rate. How? By natural means. Famine and sickness.*[102]

---

[101] Mark P. Mattson, "Hormesis Defined," *Ageing Research Reviews* 7, no. 1 (January 2008): 1–7, doi:10.1016/j.arr.2007.08.007.

[102] "Robert McNamara Quote," *A-Z Quotes*, accessed July 11, 2017, http://www.azquotes.com/quote/1268585.

McNamara is wrong. Hormesis informs us that chronic stress causes population ***explosion*** (with increased morbidity and mortality) — not population ***reduction***.

Similarly, Bill Gates is often quoted by anti-vaxers as saying and meaning:

> *Vaccines are the best way to depopulate...*

Again, mild hormetic poisoning actually causes population increase, not "depopulation". The great population increases of the impoverished and polluted are renowned.

Market reality

Little difference exists between the "benefit" of hormetic poisoning and the damage from chronic poisoning. Thayer (2005):

> *The mechanism of one family of... dose response curves has been thoroughly explored, and the details are not consistent with a beneficial effect.*[103]

Definitions of hormesis are driven by marketeers who want consumers to view temporary toxic highs as beneficial. They need to see hormesis related to "vitality", "potential of life", and "beneficial effects".

Apologists for pollution even argue that nuclear radiation adds spring to your step. Arsenic has been sold as a stimulating "tonic", competing with cocaine-laden, and now caffeine-laden, *Coca Cola*. Arsenic tonic is still given to race horses.

---

[103] KA Thayer, R Melnick, K Burns, D Davis, J Huff, "Our Stolen Future: Irresponsible Flaws in Proposed Regulatory Application of Hormesis," *Environmental Health Perspectives*, 2005, http://www.ourstolenfuture.org/NewScience/regulatory/2005/2005-0615thayeretal.htm.

Terms that are commonly used to describe hormetic effects, must be corrected. "Vitality" should be replaced with "mania" or "high" to remind us of the real nature of hormesis.

The hormetic effect is a drug effect, a destabilizing illusion eventually requiring correction (depression, hangover, migraines, etc).

The pharmaceutical industry is vested in hormesis as it persuades that poison pills produce beneficial effects. Manipulation of hormetic paradigms maintain disinfo mysteries wherever gene or germ theories fail.

BY-PHASIC DISEASES

Hormesis describes bi-phasic dose symptoms. That is, there is a hormetic threshold around which ***opposite diseases*** occur within a syndrome. This is a known dynamic.

I will argue DUS causation for several bi-phasic diseases.

ADHD vs ASD (as hormetic opposites)

Microcephaly, ADHD, and ASD are often comorbid. Romero (2015):

> *The symptoms of autism spectrum disorders and ADHD overlap.* [104]

Malinger (2003):

---

[104] Maria Carmen Carrascosa-Romero and Carlos De Cabo-De La Vega, "The Comorbidity of ADHD and Autism Spectrum Disorders (ASDs) in Community Preschoolers," 2015, doi:10.5772/61400.

> *The smaller the head circumference, the higher the chances of associated mental retardation.* [105]

ADHD is a neurodevelopmental disorder, characterized by attention deficit, excessive activity, and/or difficulty controlling behavior not appropriate for age.

ASD is described as neurological damage with comorbidities. My hormesis graph asserts a toxicology of ADHD and ASD:

---

[105] Gustavo Malinger, Dorit Lev, and Tally Lerman-Sagie, "Assessment of Fetal Intracranial Pathologies First Demonstrated Late in Pregnancy: Cell Proliferation Disorders," *Reproductive Biology and Endocrinology* 1 (2003): 110, doi:10.1186/1477-7827-1-110.

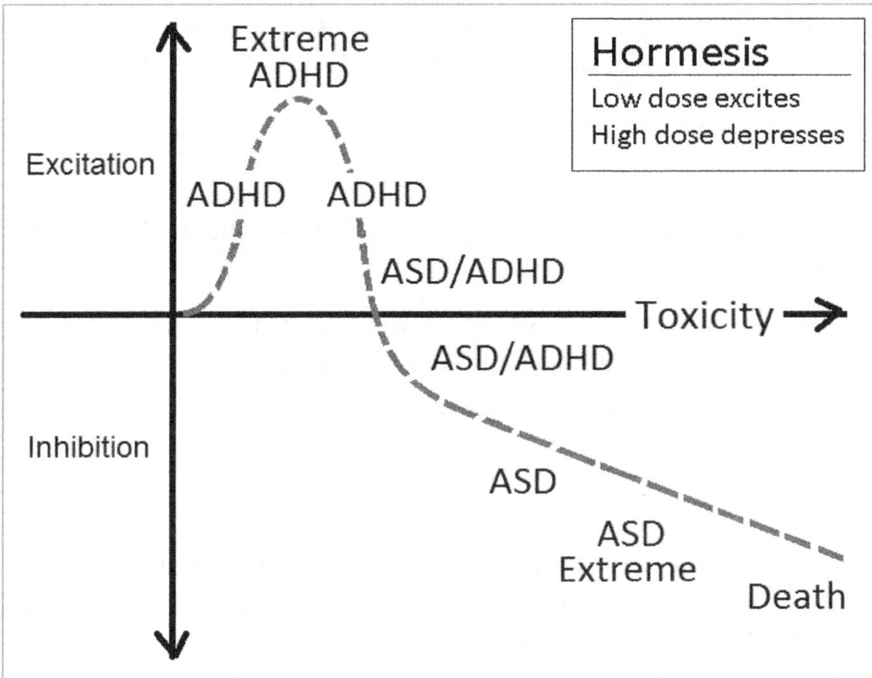

Life expectancy for ADHD and ASD children is substantially lower than the norm, with a 200% higher risk of early death for ADHD children,[106] and, as is well known, much worse for ASD children.

Microcephaly vs MACROcephaly (as hormetic opposites)

The epidemic of NE Brazil publicized the symptoms of microcephaly, but nothing was said about MACROcephaly. Both are often comorbid with autism.

---

[106] Søren Dalsgaard et al., "Mortality in Children, Adolescents, and Adults with Attention Deficit Hyperactivity Disorder: A Nationwide Cohort Study," *The Lancet* 385, no. 9983 (May 30, 2015): 2190–96, doi:10.1016/S0140-6736(14)61684-6.

MACROcephaly can continue growth for several years before becoming obvious enough for a diagnosis. Lainhart (1997):

> *Rates of head growth may be abnormal in early and middle childhood in some (37%) children with autism.*[107]

The 37% includes microcephaly and MACROcephaly, mostly the latter.

Fombonne (1999)[108] found microcephaly at 15% and MACROcephaly at 20% in autistic children, which approximates Lainhart's 37%. This can be used to estimate prevalence in the general population.

Postulates

Present-era, microcephaly and MACROcephaly are both initiated by DUS damage as hormetic opposites. Microcephaly is a cautious halt of cell division, or a stunting of vital processes, or just the result of damage. MACROcephaly is adaptive overgrowth following damage. Too much damage and MACROcephaly is not possible — only microcephaly would be possible.

MACROcephaly is often detected later than congenital microcephaly. Lainhart (1997) and Fombonne (1999) state usually detected later, but Gillberg (2002), more definitive on this point, found congenital MACROcephaly more common than microcephaly.

---

[107] J. E. Lainhart et al., "MACROcephaly in Children and Adults with Autism," *Journal of the American Academy of Child and Adolescent Psychiatry* 36, no. 2 (February 1997): 282–90, doi:10.1097/00004583-199702000-00019.

[108] E. Fombonne et al., "Microcephaly and MACROcephaly in Autism," *Journal of Autism and Developmental Disorders* 29, no. 2 (April 1999): 113–19.

These dichotomous cephalies within DUS Syndrome vary according to dose.

Microcephaly is the result of a metabolism shutdown, a growth shutdown, a cell division shutdown, due to radiation damage. Cell division is a most vulnerable process, unlikely to proceed at a normal pace under the threat of radiation.

It makes sense that developmental delays and neurological disorders are usually comorbid with congenital microcephaly and MACROcephaly.

L. Kathleen Mahan, an expert in clinical pediatrics, notes their coexistence:

> *...early microcephaly followed by MACROcephaly at 1 year.*[109]

Ivanovic (2004) finds both as indicators of brain pathology.

> *...microcephaly and MACROcephaly are considered reliable indicators of brain pathology... head circumference values below the mean are associated with an increased incidence of lower intellectual abilities...*[110]

Consider the NE Brazil timeline report. *The Network* measured head size, but only reported microcephaly via Soares (2016). Likely, an even greater MACROcephaly epidemic could have been

---

[109] L Kathleen Mahan, "Nutrition in Autism [Micro-MACROcephaly]," accessed June 20, 2016, http://210.0.231.168/Files/AlwaysOnLearning/1280Nutrition_in_Austism.pdf.

[110] Daniza M. Ivanovic et al., "Head Size and Intelligence, Learning, Nutritional Status and Brain Development. Head, IQ, Learning, Nutrition and Brain," *Neuropsychologia* 42, no. 8 (2004): 1118–31, doi:10.1016/j.neuropsychologia.2003.11.022.

reported, as the study was tasked three years after the microcephaly epidemic began, time enough for the recognition of early and late MACROcephaly.

HORMETIC SPECTRUM

In Brazil, microcephaly was diagnosed at birth with comorbid disorders (ocular, hearing, etc.) but these were not included in the reported timeline. We should expect those comorbidities, and others such as ASD, ADHD, heart disease and MACROcephaly.

In general, "The Autistic Spectrum Disorders Report" (2009) discusses a wide variety of disorders associated with ASD that include both microcephaly and MACROcephaly:

> *The most frequent Central Nervous System (CNS) disorders reported were Microcephaly, Cerebral Palsy, Chiari Malformation and Absent or Thin Corpus Callosum. The number of* ***microcephaly*** *(small head) cases was interesting since recent studies have suggested an increased rate of* ***MACROcephaly*** *(large head) in autism.*[111]

Grether (2009):

> *...the initiating process leading to ASD typically begins during fetal development...*[112]

---

[111] The National Birth Defects Registry, "Autistic Spectrum Disorders Report" (Birth Defect Research for Children, 2009), http://www.birthdefects.org/wp-content/uploads/2014/02/ASD-Report-2009.pdf.

[112] Judith K. Grether et al., "Antenatal Ultrasound and Risk of Autism Spectrum Disorders," *Journal of Autism and Developmental Disorders* 40, no. 2 (September 1, 2009): 238–45, doi:10.1007/s10803-009-0859-4.

Geschwind (2009) states that prenatal “overgrowth” exculpates vaccine causation. While true, this is good evidence for prenatal DUS:

> *Brain Overgrowth and Macrocephaly: ...brain “overgrowth” in ASD... clearly implicates an early neurodevelopmental process [prenatal) which] argues against vaccine or postnatal toxin involvement, as the [initial] process underlying brain overgrowth [is likely] prior to these purported exposures.*[113]

Normal head size, as expected genetically, might even be uncommon. The unusual case of Normalcy would be the result of two unlikely possibilities, 1) avoidance of prenatal medical radiation sessions, or 2) good luck during those sessions.

---

[113] Daniel H. Geschwind, “Advances in Autism,” *Annual Review of Medicine* 60 (2009): 367–80, doi:10.1146/annurev.med.60.053107.121225.

Autism is generally more damaging than ADHD and Asperger. See my graphic rendition of congenital OFC (Occipital Frontal Circumference) data from Gillberg (2002).[114] Asperger syndrome is high-functioning autism, though technically these are separate diagnoses.

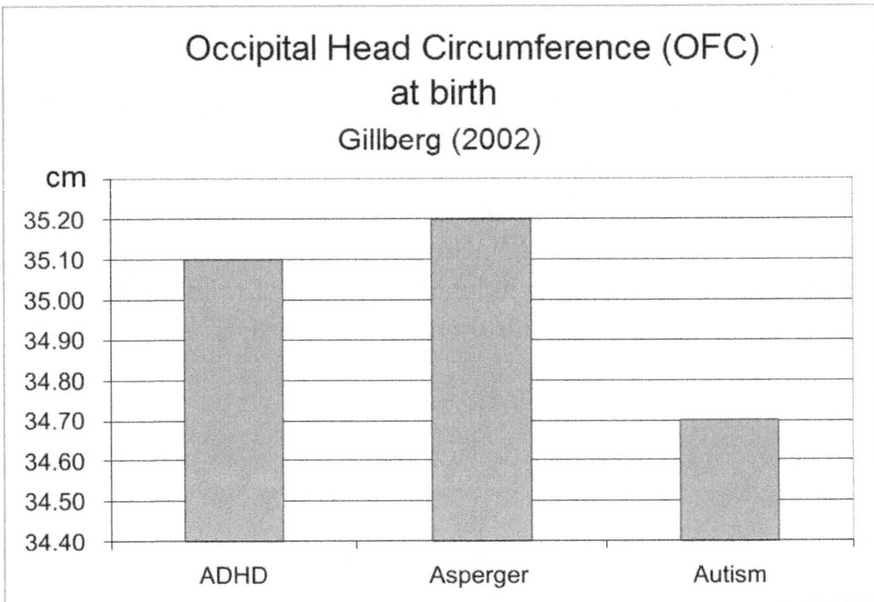

[114] Christopher Gillberg and Linda De Souza, "Head Circumference in Autism, Asperger Syndrome, and ADHD: A Comparative Study," *Developmental Medicine & Child Neurology* 44, no. 5 (May 1, 2002): 296–300, doi:10.1111/j.1469-8749.2002.tb00814.x.

Average congenital MACROcephaly, per group, can change during childhood. See next graph.

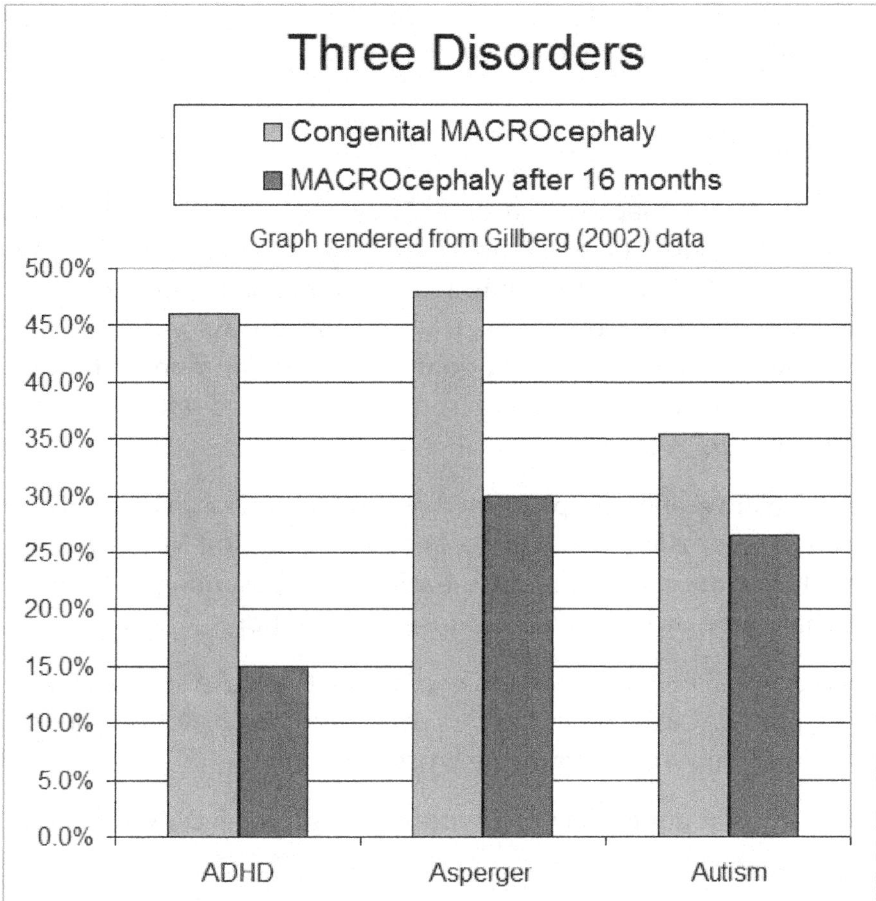

The graph represents three groups, their average change from MACROcephaly at birth to less MACROcephaly at 16 months and older. The graph does not describe ***individual*** cases of developmental MACROcephaly (the emergence of MACROcephaly not present at birth). Gillberg, however, does state that 50% of Asperger cases and about 65% of autism cases were found to be developmental MACROcephaly, when measured any time after 16 months, often several years later.

With the knowledge gained so far, we can now speculate as follows.

Diagnostic snapshots

Diagnoses are snapshots in time. They give a name to observations of bioeffects at a point in time. Gillberg (2002) and Geschwind (2009) tell us that infant microcephaly and MACROcephaly can change over time. If we reasonably assume that DUS generally initiates such conditions in the womb, months before they are diagnosed, we can reasonably surmise how those conditions change over time.

Six timeline graphs are presented below that approximate and extend the aforesaid discussions of microcephaly and MACROcephaly. I introduce and annotate each graph, assuming that both cephaly types are survival responses to radiation.

Microcephaly is presumed to generally be the more severe condition, and MACROcephaly the less severe condition. Some types of microcephaly would simply be gross destruction.

Each subsequent graph represents higher prenatal DUS exposure.

Graph #1: Low exposure

MACROcephaly develops prenatally or when the child is birthed out its toxic radiative womb. In either case, the fetus has grown large enough to be less vulnerable to DUS radiation. The child eventually attains a normal head size after an early period of catch-up, overshoot, and adaptive MACROcephaly anywhere between 1 to 7 years following birth. No microcephaly.

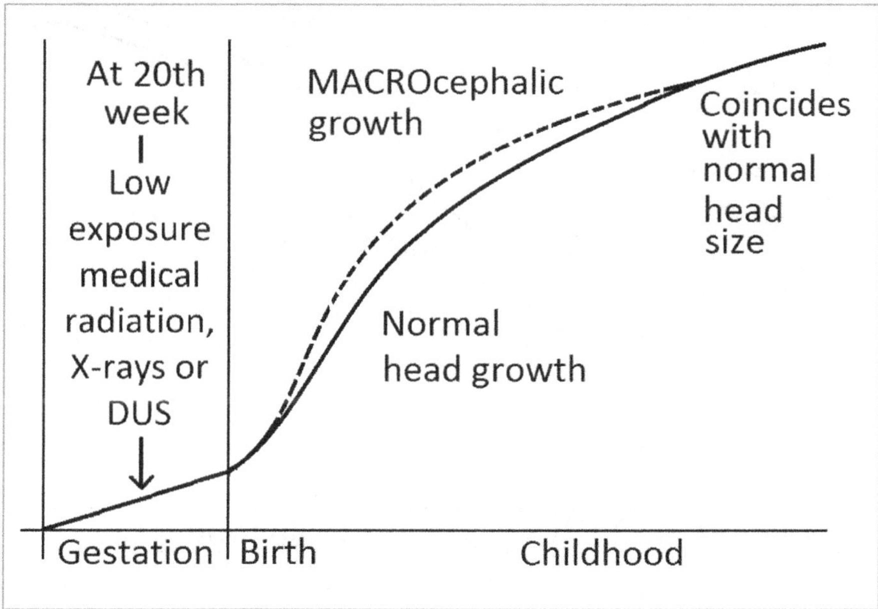

Graph #2: Medium exposure

The child maintains sustained MACROcephaly from birth, and in some cases this could begin in the womb at 20 weeks gestation. No microcephaly.

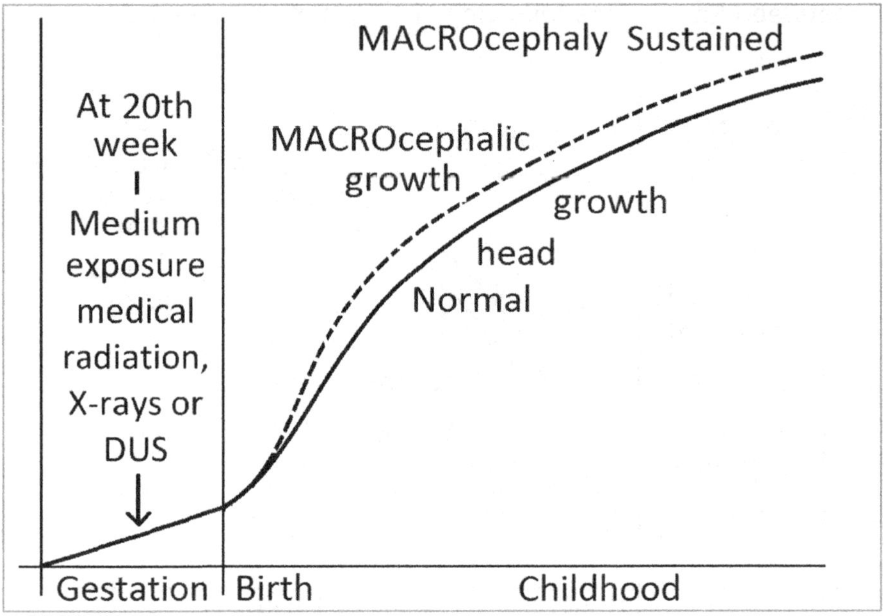

Graph #3: High exposure

IUGR/microcephaly begins during gestation, with MACROcephaly following after birth to eventually catch up to normal head size, then surpassing and attaining a diagnosis of late MACROcephaly.

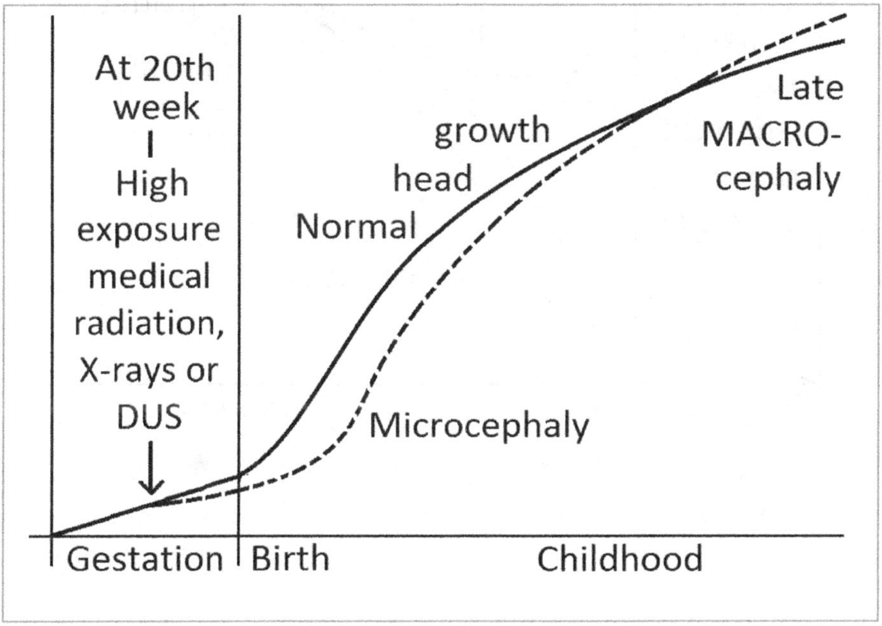

Graph #4: Higher exposure

IUGR and microcephaly begins during gestation and over-growth catches up to normal head size.

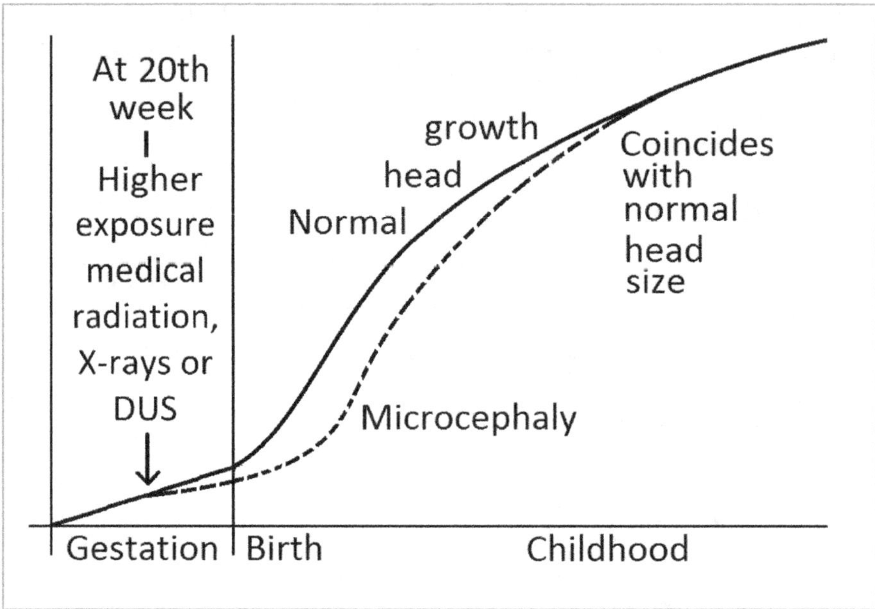

Graph #5: Very High exposure

IUGR/microcephaly begins during gestation and overgrowth catches up to sustained sub-normal head size.

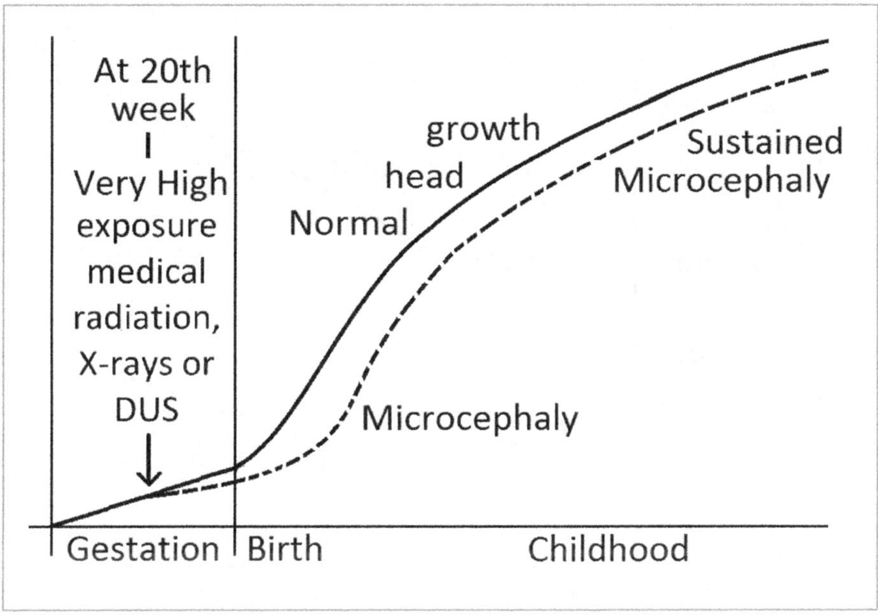

Graph #6: Extreme exposure

IUGR and microcephaly begin during gestation, continuing as sustained microcephaly or as proportional microcephaly with small body size.

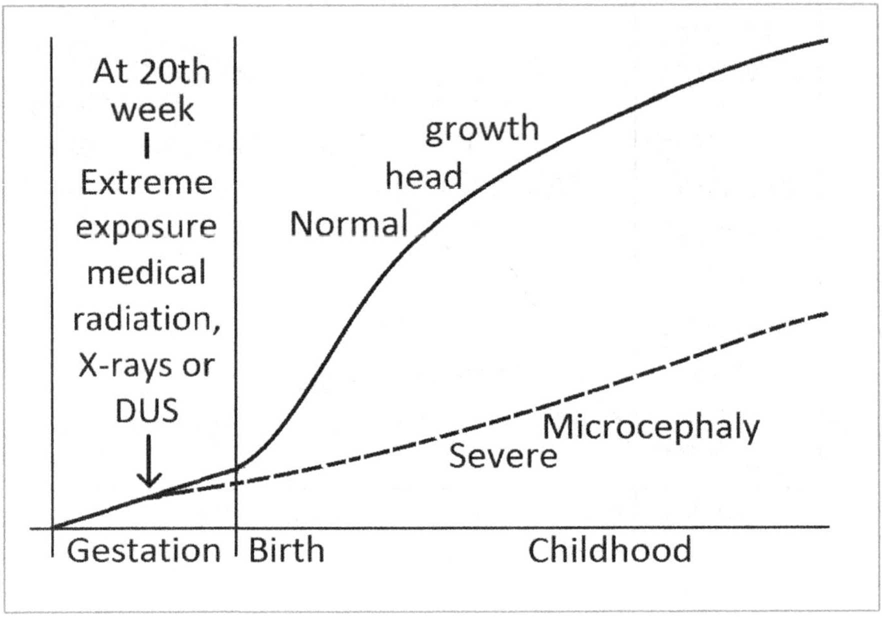

Those are a few general scenarios. Infinite variations exist, for example, if a DUS transducer were focused excessively on the brain rather than the body — then that would be isolated cephaly. If wider damage occurs, then the cephaly would be syndromic. Syndromic is known to be the most common type, and that happens to be the typical prenatal DUS exposure scenario, a wide application of ultrasound to the fetus, with the worst tragedy being the result of exposure to the fetal brain, eyes, ears, heart, etc.

Evidence of DUS damage: Microcephaly, MACROcephaly, Proportional microcephaly, Proportional MACROcephaly, and other brain/head distortions (cone head, flat head, etc).

Another scenario

The MACROcephalic overgrowth process would not necessarily attain the status of MACROcephaly because it is starting from a state of microcephaly. At birth, then, there could emerge microcephaly, normality or MACROcephaly, yet all are a different snapshot view (diagnosis) of the same process.

Prenatal microcephaly could exist within a state of MACROcephalic growth.

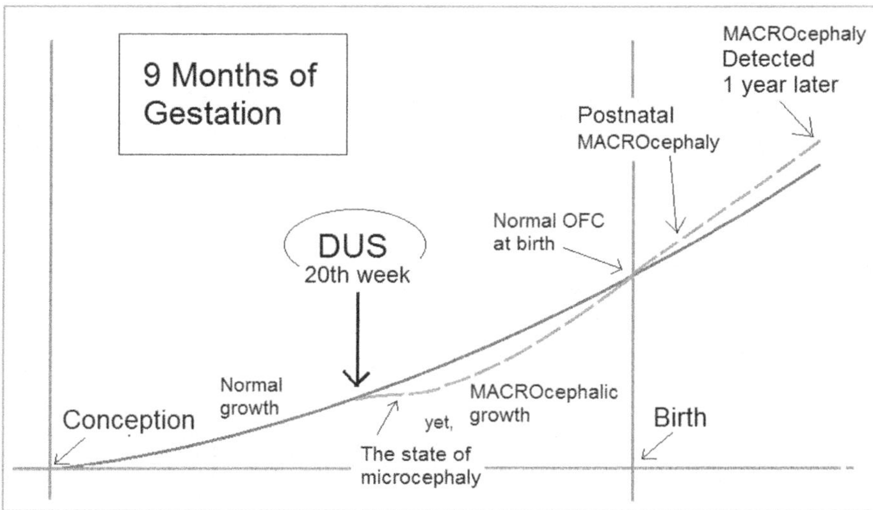

10 | Proportional MACROcephaly

Occult epidemic

Interim summary

Contrasting with earlier studies, Gillberg (2002) found 46% congenital MACROcephaly in ADHD neonates.

Gillberg's finds that MACROcephaly is generally overlooked at birth.

I appreciate this important study, as I nevertheless bring a critical review.

PROPORTIONAL MACROCEPHALY

Gillberg **excluded** Proportional MACROcephaly by definition. This is a MACROcephaly type where the head and body are both abnormally large (as mentioned earlier).

Gillberg's definitions require that the head must be larger than the body to qualify as MACROcephaly. Thereby, it limits perception of the maximum prevalence of MACROcephaly within the U.S. autistic and general populations.

Gillberg (2002) admits this limitation, while obfuscating its extent, as demonstrated by the following analysis table.

Analysis of Gillberg (2002) Two Definition of MACROcephaly: Genuine and Relative	
Gillberg (2002), extracts	**JW comments**
Definition #1, Genuine MACROcephaly In one paragraph, one definition	
Genuine MACROcephalus was considered to be present	"Genuine MACRO-cephalus"
in children whose OFC surpassed the age and sex normative data by 2SDs or more	Must be unusually large heads (head circumference (OFC))
and	and...
whose height and weight were both 1SD or more under that expected on the basis of the OFC.	Body size (height and weight) must be proportionally less than head circumference (OFC). This is a strict exclusion of Proportional MACROcephaly cases.
It was argued that genuine macrocephalus would not be an appropriate label for children with large heads proportional to overall body size.	This explains why Proportional MACROcephaly is excluded from this Definition #1.

Definition #2, Relative Macrocephaly **In one paragraph, two sub-definitions**	
Relative macrocephalus was considered to be present	"Relative MACROcephalus"
(1) in children whose OFC surpassed the age and sex normative values by 2SDs or more	Sub-definition (a): Must have unusually large heads (head circumference, OFC)
and	and...
whose height or weight, but not both, was 1SD or more under that expected on the basis of the OFC,	Body size (height or weight) must be Proportionally less than head circumference (OFC). This definition thus also excludes Proportional MACROcephaly cases, but less strictly.
and	and...
(2) in patients whose OFC was above the age and sex normative values and whose height was 1.5SDs or more below the level expected on the basis of the OFC.	Sub-definition (b): "children" are now "patients", thereby throwing the reader off. Body size (height) must be Proportionally less than head circumference (OFC), thus again excluding

	Proportional MACROcephaly.
[Explanation missing]	No explanation here for why Proportional MACROcephaly is excluded (though provided in Definition #1.)

Discussion

Gillberg (2002) studied three disorder groups (ADHD, Asperger, and ASD), and found a high incidence of MACROcephaly.

Proportional MACROcephaly cases were excluded by all definitions. The data was found but not presented.

The explanation of the limitation should have been applied to both definitions (once above both definitions or added to each definition). Yet it was tucked into Definition #1 as if it only applied to Definition #1. The reader could assume incorrectly that the complex and strangely worded Definition #2 handles the limitation of Definition #1.

Obfuscated is the exclusion of a MACROcephaly type that would include a large (proportional) body. Obfuscated is the exclusion of relevant discussion.

Large head/body would be expected from prenatal medical radiation, whenever it mildly damages the head and body. The study determined the relevant data, and so it should have presented it via a Definition #3, "Proportional cases". It could avoid over-diagnosing large body children by discounting the norm. Failing that, then a more thorough explanation is necessary for this important topic, but there is no such explanation.

How could essential norms be determined if growth weight is declining every year (see previous topic, "Weight reduction")? This requires discussion.

The authors may say this is all an innocent clumsiness or insurmountable problem, but the topic is too important, too close to the core of the study to get wrong or omit discussion. The issue appears skated as a political solution.

Considerations

“Proportional MACROcephaly” exists as a widespread pathological condition.

Epidemic MACROcephaly is apparent by simply looking around at the present-day child population and wondering why public conversations are devoid of discussion re a present U.S. MACROcephaly epidemic, more prevalent than microcephaly. Ditto for NE Brazil. The disinterest in true MACROcephaly prevalence would be an understandable prerequisite for publication.

It is possible that MACROcephaly, initiated in the womb from microcephaly, could still be smaller than normal head circumference at birth. It is even possible that MACROcephaly could coexist with a body proportionally larger than the head.

Officially, there are dichotomous disorders of “microcephaly and MACROcephaly”, but consider the dichotomous disorders of “IUGR and [what?]”

The dichotomy could be “IUGR and IUGE”, where IUGE would be the acronym for Intra-Uterine Growth Expansion. Medicos do refer to “large body size”, though not often as a disorder. IUGE could exist as a hormetic disorder, or as a synonym for MACROcephalic growth.

Continue with

Part B

The publish date for Part B depends on the public interest in Part A. Request notification at www.harvoa.org/contact

—Syndrome Revisions—

- DUS Syndrome
- Congenital Rubella Syndrome
- Chorioamnionitis

—Northeast Brazil—

- Microcephaly in NE Brazil
- DUS the Teratogen
- Fetal Echocardiography
- *The Network*

Part C

—Northeast Brazil (continued)—

- The Perfect Population Study

- The Mattos Interview

—Studies—

- Brasil (2016): Study
- Columbia: DUS Market Push
- Twin Studies
- Inappropriate Studies
- Biased Studies
- The First Zika Study

—*The Hypothesis* Applied—

- Discussion with a Psych PhD
- Vaxxed: Film Review
- Vaxxed: Addenda
- Improving Anti-Vax Arguments
- Relationships
- To DUS or Not to DUS

—A Hero—

- Ruo Feng: Biography

Other books by Jim West

[DUS Book 1]
Ultrasound: A New Bibliography; The Chinese Studies
[Human empirical studies]

[Polio Book]
DDT/Polio
Original research into the toxicology of polio, with graphs, tables, and text. This challenges poliovirus and virology, finds hidden arcana, constructs a toxicological concept for Franklin Delano Roosevelt's polio, and presents historical epidemiological timelines and dose/response studies.

—Appendices—

A | Proof Tables

The Hypothesis stated in a proof table	
Statement	**Reason/Reference**
DUS caused the microcephaly epidemic in NE Brazil	Thesis
"Anything that impairs growth and integrity of the brain from the time of its early development to the end of the postnatal growth period may lead to microcephaly."	Stevenson (2005)[115]
"Microcephaly may result from any insult that disturbs early brain growth..."	Ashwal (2009)
DUS is capable of damaging all fetal organs, especially the neurological system, including the brain. This fulfills Ashwal's "any insult".	See chapter "Confirmation" herein.

[115] Roger E. Stevenson, Dir and Columbia, *Human Malformations and Related Anomalies*, 473.

DUS causes growth restriction, a syndrome that includes microcephaly. DUS usually occurs in the early second trimester. This fulfills "disturbs early brain growth" (above).	See chapter "Growth Restriction" herein.
Microcephaly comorbidity is evidently DUS damage.	See chapter "DUS Syndrome" herein.
Modern Medicine avoids the topic of DUS causation and discourages research. It ignores studies that indict DUS. This indicates conflict of interest and the hiding of DUS damage.	See Chapter 6 of DUS Book 1 for authoritative but repressive and repressed statements re DUS causation.
High-intensity DUS is able to cause microcephaly.	Sub-conclusion
Unique, unprecedented, high-intensity DUS correlates with time and location for the epidemic of NE Brazil. The epidemic data itself is the "Smoking Gun", serving as an excellent population study of modern high exposure DUS.	Mattos (2015) Soares (2016) See Part B.
All other environmental agents (as evaluated by both Modern Medicine and environmentalists) fail to explain causation for the epidemic.	

Modern Medicine did not rigorously study environmental agents for microcephaly causation, such as chemicals and strictly so, medical radiation. Given the evidence for medical radiation, strict avoidance of the radiation topic indicates conflict of interest, heavy bias and the probable hiding of DUS damage.	Rasmussen (2016), where environmental agents are briefly mentioned. Soares (2016) criticizes the omission of environmental causation.[116]
All environmental agents fail, except the rigorously avoided item, radiation.	Sub-conclusion
The mainstream theory is Zika virus. Infection fails to explain causation.	Rasmussen (2016) admits, "There is no smoking gun."
Zika virus paradigm is unproven.	Sub-conclusion
WHO admits maniacal bias by declaring Zika virus "guilty until proven innocent."	Dr. Anthony Costello, high official at WHO.
Zika causation bias is maniacal	Sub-conclusion
The original discovery of Zika virus in 1947 is patently false.	See Part C, "Virus causation".

[116] Soares de Araújo et al., "Microcephaly in Northeastern Brazil."

Zika virus is a false paradigm	Sub-conclusion
The most obvious cause, medical radiation, is not mentioned, out of conflict of interest.	Radiation avoidance
X-ray and DUS share similar patterns of comorbidity.	9 | DUS Syndrome
However, there is no evidence of X-rays applied at extraordinary exposure levels in NE Brazil. Even Modern Medicine generally warns against prenatal X-rays.	Mattos (2015)
X-ray causation fails.	Sub-conclusion
Mere suspicion of microcephaly cases brings advice for "serial ultrasonography". This indicates corruption or naiveté.	Brasil (2016)[117]
Genetic causation science is merely "associative".	Kohn (2003)
Genetic causation fails.	Sub-conclusion
DUS thesis succeeds.	Conclusion

[117] Brasil et al., "Zika Virus Infection in Pregnant Women in Rio de Janeiro — Preliminary Report."

Proof Table by Sub-Conclusions Only	
Statement	**Reason/Reference**
DUS caused the microcephaly epidemic in NE Brazil	Thesis
High-intensity DUS is able to cause microcephaly.	
All environmental agents fail, except the most rigorously avoided suspect, radiation.	
Zika virus paradigm is admittedly unproven for microcephaly causation.	
Mainstream Zika bias is maniacal.	
Zika virus is a false paradigm.	
X ray causation fails.	
Genetic causation fails.	
Much more evidence exists for DUS than for any other agent.	
DUS thesis succeeds.	Conclusion

B | Webb (2016) and AIUM

Webb (2016) is a human population study, with lead author, Pierre Mourad, PhD. It is titled:

Severity of ASD symptoms and their correlation with the presence of copy number variations and exposure to first trimester ultrasound[118]

Abstract [Extract]

> *Casanova proposed a triple hit hypothesis where the convergence of three factors (1) the brain of a genetically at risk individual is (2) exposed during a time of critical neurodevelopment to (3) an exogenous stressor, may contribute to the incidence of ASD. First, the stressor occurs during a critical period of brain development. In ASD, it has been proposed that this insult occurs early in gestation (e.g. 1st or 2nd trimester)...*
>
> *We found that male children with ASD, copy number variations (CNVs), and exposure to first trimester ultrasound*

---

[118] Jane Webb et al., "Severity of ASD Symptoms and Their Correlation with the Presence of Copy Number Variations and Exposure to First Trimester Ultrasound."

had significantly decreased non-verbal IQ and increased repetitive behaviors [compared] to male children with ASD, with CNVs, and no ultrasound.

AIUM responds against Webb (2016)

September 7, 2016

AIUM Bioeffects Committee Statement on Paper[119]

The study did not test the original hypothesis because it did not include a comparison control group, namely, a sibling comparison group, and this was a significant flaw in the study. The occurrence of ultrasound in the first trimester was determined solely by parental recall. No information was provided on the details of the ultrasound exposure, including the indication for the ultrasound, type of ultrasound (abdominal or transvaginal), exposure duration, exposure during other trimesters, or imaging modality. Furthermore, the study did not test for numerous possible confounding factors. The authors also did not perform a Bonferroni correction for multiple comparisons, which would be appropriate for a confirmatory study establishing causal connections. The results are not significant at the 5% level with a Bonferroni correction. In the absence of such a correction, the authors should have explicitly stated that this was an exploratory analysis designed to uncover correlations that need to be confirmed in a future study. In summary, the results of the study do not demonstrate a causal link between ultrasound and autism. Ultrasound examinations can be safely performed by educated and credentialed sonographers and clinicians

---

[119] AIUM Bioeffects Committee, "AIUM Responds to Autism Study," *AIUM*, September 7, 2016, http://www.aium.org/soundWaves/article.aspx?aId=965&iId=20160907.

when medically indicated and when the ALARA (as low as reasonable achievable) principle is followed.

Pierre Mourad replies to AIUM

...We sought to determine if exposure to diagnostic ultrasound might correlate with autism spectrum disorder (ASD) severity (not incidence) framed as a modified triple hit hypothesis (Casanova 2007). Specifically, we asked, might the severity of ASD symptoms correlate with (1) ultrasound exposure (2) during the first trimester of pregnancy in fetuses with a (3) genetic predisposition to ASD.

Among our results, we observed in all ASD children with known copy number variations (CNVs, a specific class of genetic defect associated with ASD and other neurodevelopmental disorders) and exposure to ultrasound during the first trimester that non-verbal IQ determined clinically was statistically significantly lower than for those not exposed to ultrasound, with, in addition, trends towards increased repetitive behaviors determined clinically and increased impaired adaptive behaviors via parent report... Moreover, male ASD children with CNVs and first trimester exposure relative to those not exposed to first trimester ultrasound also had lower non-verbal IQ determined clinically as well as an increase in repetitive behaviors determined clinically, along with consistent trends in verbal IQ determined clinically and repetitive behaviors via parent report... We further note that in post-hoc analysis we did not find a correlation between ASD symptom severity, presence of CNVs and exposure to ultrasound during either of the second or third trimesters...

Our paper contained statistical analysis that included explicitly documented and robust tests for the effects of an extensive list of confounding factors on our results... As we reported, Olsen et al (1997) found that maternal memory for pregnancy related events is relatively good; albeit, we also noted that the parental memory for identifying timing of ultrasound, particularly when occurring at 10-14 weeks, may create random error in reporting. Because of this concern we performed analysis reported in the paper that showed that our results were insensitive to this potential error. Also, as stated in the paper, we could not study incidence of ASD, as this data set did not include sufficient medical information about any plausible control population, such as individuals without ASD or siblings of children with ASD. Finally, we did not infer a causal link between ASD symptom severity and exposure to first trimester ultrasound in our paper...

In our manuscript and within this response, we call for support for FDA guidelines that seek to limit diagnostic ultrasound for obstetrical care to those cases with medical need.

Given the documentation by those in the AIUM community of non-medical use of diagnostic ultrasound, insufficient attention to ALARA by medical providers, among other concerns (e.g., Abramowicz, 2013) our recommendations are also in direct line with AIUM statements. We also call for more research on possible gene by environment interactions that include ultrasound exposure...

In short, we found a statistically significant correlation between ASD severity and the presence of CNVs and exposure to first-trimester ultrasound. Our results support, in our view, FDA and AIUM guidelines for the use of ultrasound during obstetrical care as well as motivates further biological and biophysical research.

My notes

AIUM ignored Mourad's reply.

CNV is the acronym for Copy Number Variation, a type of structural variation of DNA. CNVs here represent vulnerabilities, not necessarily inherited. I suggest that CNVs themselves could also have been caused by DUS, and that puts an additional twist to Webb (2016), perhaps revealing the political ingenuity of its design in a world where genetic causation is favored for funding and publication.

Webb (2016) is politically correct in that it maintains the possibility of genetic vulnerability.

Webb provides an answer to this big question from Dodge (2011):

> *Why... are chromosome anomalies, congenital anomalies, minor congenital anomalies, and CNVs so frequent in autism?* [120]

Clarification of Mourad's reply Table by Jim West	
Both column's are Mourad's text	
Among our results, we observed	
in all ASD children with known copy number variations	(CNVs, a specific class of genetic defect associated with ASD and

---

[120] Kenneth A. Dodge and Michael Rutter, *Gene-Environment Interactions in Developmental Psychopathology* (Guilford Press, 2011).

	other neurodevelopmental disorders)
and	
exposure to ultrasound during the first trimester	
that	
non-verbal IQ (determined clinically)	[Parentheses added]
was statistically significantly lower	
than	
for those not exposed to ultrasound,	
with	["in addition" deleted]
trends towards increased repetitive behaviors... and increased impaired adaptive behaviors...	
Moreover...	[Furthermore, other defect variants were found correlated with ultrasound]

C | Infectious Illusions

Microbial infection exists, however, as disease causation it is overplayed by Mainstream Medicine.

Here are several alternative explanations for infection.

THE SIMPLE ILLUSION (OF INFECTION)

Dr. Stefan Lanka is renowned for his general critique of germ theory. In 2000, during his lecture at HEAL-NYC (Michael Ellner's group), he responded to parents who had observed "spreading infection" among children at chickenpox parties. Lanka stated that infection did not really happen with regard to the observed transmission of symptoms. "Infection" was an illusion perpetuated by propaganda during a period of actual toxicological symptoms.

His was a fine answer, but the audience rebelled, as chickenpox infection seemed very real in the context of their own experience with their children.

The rebellion was supported over a decade later by Dr. Suzanne Humphries, her defense of germ theory against John Wantling, on her Facebook page. John then asked me for rebuttal ideas:

> *Explain to me why children go to a chicken pox party and at around the same time most if not all get the same symptoms.*

And thus this article where I extend Lanka's brief answer.

Though Humphries is much better than her professional peers, by needlessly embracing infection paradigms, she provides argument handles to her mainstream opponents.

The concept of infection is motivated into existence by a pervasive conflict of interest: Medicos often claim infection without direct evidence, thereby enabling vaccine sales, profitable toxicological and medical complications, and protection for polluting industries that dominate the medical industry.

The Power of Suggested Infection

When a group is poisoned by air pollution flu, there must be a first person who succumbs to symptoms before anyone else, then others follow like popping popcorn. The cause is likely an accumulation or acute exposure to environmental assaults along with differences in inherited defense behaviors. Those who show symptoms first are considered to be chemically sensitive. These people "suggest" the good idea of an appropriate disease response (symptoms) to others in the group, like a yawn or sneeze, with no contact required. There is no reason why we should all have the same responses ready in our minds, when we can help each other out with good ideas.

The Popcorn Analogy

For a moment, pretend that popping corn is a disease, spreading like an epidemic infection, first a few then many. Popping corn looks like an active infection if the popper machine's heat source were not so obvious. Clearly the cause is environmental.

Medicos would profit if they could claim that unpopped corn is immune to the popping germ, immune to popping infection. Medicos could sell vaccines that prevent each kernel from popping. They

COULD ALSO MANDATE THE EXCLUSIVE USE OF GENETICALLY MODIFIED CORN THAT WOULD NOT SUCCUMB TO POPPING DISEASE.

Germ Theory: Toxicological Avoidance

Looking at a hot air popcorn popper...

If we were required to ignore heating elements, and also required to explain popcorn causation, we would have two choices. 1) Infection from one kernel to the other, or, 2) Innate kernel vulnerability to popability. These are analogous to germ or genetic causation paradigms.

That is medical reality, enforced toxicological blindness, yet required to explain disease.

Influential Hormones

This interpretation is related to and combined with, the power of suggestion, though here the suggestion is transmitted not by body language or acoustic or written words. Consider pheromones creating the illusion of germ infection.

Wikipedia [bolding is mine]:

> *A pheromone (from Greek... phero "to bear" and hormone... "impetus") is a secreted or excreted* ***chemical*** *factor that* ***triggers a social response...*** *Pheromones are chemicals capable of acting outside the body of the secreting individual to impact the behavior of the receiving individual. There are alarm pheromones, food trail pheromones, sex pheromones, and many others that affect behavior or physiology. Pheromones are used from basic unicellular prokaryotes to complex multicellular eukaryotes. Their use among insects has been particularly well documented. In addition, some vertebrates and plants communicate by using pheromones.*

Such communication would go far beyond pheromones.

Many of the observed effects of a 'virus', found in a lab or at a chickenpox party, are likely due to such inter-intra-cellular communications. Hormones have similar memory and manipulative capabilities as do the regular nervous system, however, they are slower, yet they can zing through the body interactively.[121]

Hormonal substances can flow with the body's liquids. The regular nervous system also uses hormones as neurotransmitters etc. Hormonal molecules happen to be at physical sizes similar to "viruses", so lab filterable properties would be similar for macromolecules such as hormones, and "viruses".

Two examples

Lab scenario

In a laboratory, a traumatized hormone could perpetuate "disease" (inflammatory responses) when injected from a diseased life into a healthy life. The healthy would see the traumatized hormonal context in the injection as evidence of a dangerous disease, pickup those warning signs, and perpetuate the disease behavior.

With repeated injections (passages from group to group), the disease eventually dies out, the effect of passaging disease diminishes.

Virus passaging (from one diseased animal to another by extract injection) is a laboratory parlour trick, a "laboratory artifact" to demonstrate infection. Claus Jungeblut (1952):

---

[121] Personal communication with Wirt Atmar (deceased), professor of biology and President and co-founder of AICS Research, Inc., a third-party affiliate of Hewlett-Packard. Some of his published work resides at http://www.aics-research.com/research/index.html.

> *...the highly specialized, neurotropically fixed virus, which has been maintained in the past by intracerebral passage in rhesus monkeys, is more likely a laboratory artifact...*[122]

Technicians claim to have isolated and photographed individual viruses, yet this is rarely if ever accomplished in actuality. Officials, confident in their authority, twist the word "isolation" to mean "mixture", which in a fair world, would reveal the absurdity of their so-called science.

Social scenario

Social transmission, via skin, fluids, or mists from breath or coughing or sneezing, do transmit "disease", but disease is perpetuated cellular/hormonal behavior, cathartic and defensive behavior at a cellular level.

That social group also transmits symptoms (cathartic-defensive disease) by sharing hormones in vocal, breathing, and coughing mists, or contact. But disease is usually a good thing. The bad extreme, is when sometimes the disease response may go overboard and even may trigger a severe reaction such as the disintegration of the spinal cord, to separate the spine from the brain, as a defense. I am going out on a limb there, but that would be a rare and horrible over-reaction. Over-response diseases happen more to hyped up males due to testosterone (the do or die hormone), and thus accounts for example with autism being found five times more in male children than females due to pharma or ultrasound poisoning during gestation.

Sometimes the disease response might be inappropriate, such as tooth decay. Yet, maybe tooth decay is actually appropriate, because it communicates to the community that its time to move,

---

[122] Claus W. Jungeblut, Ph.D., Journal of Pediatrics, Vol 37, p109 (July, 1950), from, Scobey, Archives of Pediatrics (April, 1952)

to leave or change the invisibly polluted environment, and/or find an environmentally aware dentist. With infection propaganda, the industrial community is stabilized, with perception of industrial poisoning defeated.

Dangerous responses to environmental symptom triggers: Examples are the laboratory virus "passaging" routine, or anaphylactic shock in an animal. An analogy is a theater on fire. People flee and are trapped in the exits where they die or are severely maimed.

Imagine a scientist taking some of the burned and traumatized persons and injecting them into a normal theater where their screaming and flailing causes the new and naive audience repeats the panic. People would run for the exits and some would be hurt, though not as badly as in the real fire. This can be perpetuated, like passaging, from theater to theater with the next phase of traumatized people, but eventually they catch on and the effect diminishes, as does so usually happen in virus passaging.

The perfume industry functions to defeat lateral social communication, i.e., the transmission among humans of pheromone communication. There are industries that produce perfume masking additives for industrial effluents to preempt societal objections. Some of these chemicals entirely block the olfactory perceptors. These industries are a hazard to human health, and they defeat the democratic process. They defeat the natural correction processes, the social resolution processes, and natural democratic communications.

Maybe these communications should be controlled, as in our industrialized poisoned society, the hormonal screams for help are unsettling. Some of the hormones suggest unusual behavioral solutions. Fortunately, medicos routinely test for abnormal hormonal behavior under the guise of germ and gene testing, then remove offending persons by quarantine or they are attenuated by antibiotic therapies.

VARYING SUSCEPTIBILITY

When a group is poisoned by, for example, air pollution, then illness first shows as respiratory symptoms, sneezing, coughing, etc.

The group responds like popcorn, a few at first and then more, giving an illusion of a deadly popping infection within the popcorn group. It all depends on the individual kernels, their vulnerability, i.e., moisture content, wall thickness, flexibility, and heat exposure.

Popped corn is not the result of infection. It is the result of heat.

Pathogen isolated and seen through an electron microscope at 500,000X:

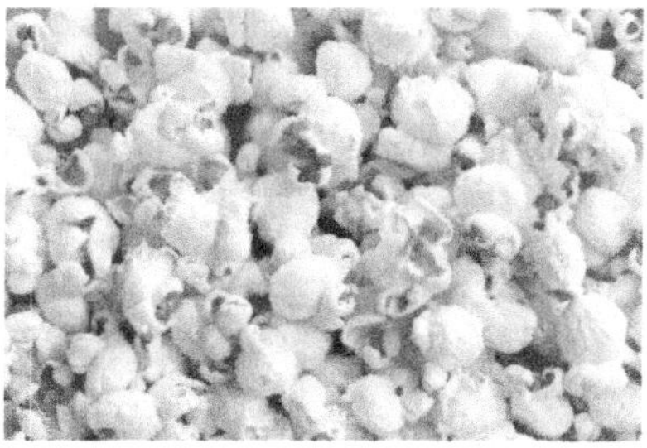

D | Pyriproxyfen

Toxicity Evaluation

Looking at Pyriproxyfen, I crunched the WHO/FAO numbers to determine years of accumulated ingestion to achieve a minimal NOAEL, taking the most negative view possible.

NOAEL = No Adverse Effect Level

NOAEL looks for any adverse bioeffect, such as a change in hormone level.

ADI is acceptable daily intake.

Pyriproxyfen Larvicide The most negative view possible		
Source for data on Pyriproxyfen, United Nations: www.fao.org/fileadmin/templates/agphome/documents/Pests_Pesticides/Specs/Pyriproxifen_2011.pdf		
Value	**Unit**	**JWest Notes**
10	mg/kg NOAEL	NOEL= No Observed Adverse Effect Level. This determined NOEL includes an uncertainty factor of 100.

0.010	g/kg NOAEL	
68	kg/typical body weight	
0.68	g/bodyweight for LD50	Lethal dose to 50% of population
0.100	ADI, max range, Pyriproxyfen/Water	accepted-daily-intake
3.00	liters (kg) water/day/person	
0.109500	g/year	probably even lower
40%	accumulated/year	probably even lower
0.044	g/year accumulated	
16	**years to NOAEL**	**Conclusion: By dosage alone, Pyriproxyfen cannot be causative for the microcephaly epidemic.**

E | Ultrasound Hazards[123]

Diagnostic ultrasound (DUS) fulfills this causation requirement by Ashwal (2009):

> ***Microcephaly may result from any insult that disturbs early brain growth...***

Ultrasound is commonly used by industry to disintegrate and blend materials, and to weld steel. Since the 1950s, ultrasound has been employed to generate "echo images" of the fetus.

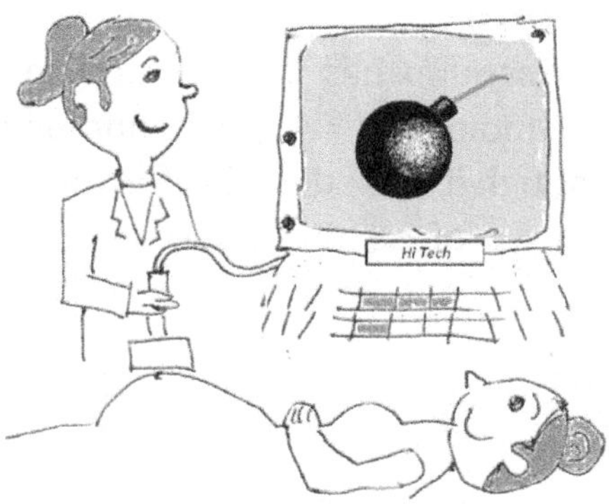

DUS is not natural sound. It is usually at a frequency of 3 to 9 megahertz, with harmonics and random sonic effects. Its fundamental frequencies are higher than the EMF carrier frequencies for the AM radio band. Human

[123] This appendix is adapted from my article published in *Townsend Letter*, April 2017.

hearing range is much lower at 20 to 20,000 hertz. DUS wave pressures can be thousands of times greater than that of the hearing pain threshold.

The physics are dramatic. Ultrasound often creates micro- and nano- size gas bubbles within liquids. This is called "cavitation" and the word was originally used to describe the destructive forces of bubbles on steel ship's propellers.

The World Health Organization's "Criteria 22", states that ultrasound cavitation can create powerful shockwaves far above the speed of sound[124] and it can create cavitational bubble collapse temperatures of thousands of degrees centigrade, greater than the surface of the sun. WHO (1982):

> *It seems reasonable to assume that effects on biological systems may be induced at least by the mechanical shock waves and high temperatures generated during the bubble collapse.*[125]

Ultrasound has largely supplanted the earlier common imaging technology, X-rays, a technology admitted to be hazardous even though it took decades for that knowledge to become public. Despite professional awareness, damaging X-ray practice continued

---

[124] Boris Krasovitski et al., "Intramembrane Cavitation as a Unifying Mechanism for Ultrasound-Induced Bioeffects," *Proceedings of the National Academy of Sciences* 108, no. 8 (February 22, 2011): 3258–63, doi:10.1073/pnas.1015771108.

[125] WHO: International Program On Chemical Safety, "Environmental Health Criteria 22: Ultrasound," 1982, http://www.inchem.org/documents/ehc/ehc/ehc22.htm.

in shoe stores, hospitals and doctors' offices. The history of medical X-ray imaging serves as a parallel to ultrasound history.[126]

DUS is now being applied to most of the entire world population during its fetal stage, and applied to nearly all pregnant women in the United States. Fearing the process of birth, women are driven towards this invasive procedure, accepting it as a standard routine.

Ina May Gaskin, legendary midwife:

> *It's easy to scare women, and it's even profitable to scare women and girls about birth.*[127]

DUS is widely declared to be "harmless" despite mothers describing on forums such as *The Thinking Moms' Revolution*, DUS-associated fetal trauma and maternal pain preceding birth to damaged children.[128] Other forums describe vaginal bleeding following DUS.[129]

Coincidentally, Torrey (1976) describes vaginal bleeding during the 2nd trimester as especially important because it is a possible marker for autism and childhood psychosis. Torrey's study was

---

[126] "Dr Robert Mendelsohn on Pregnancy and the Dangers of Ultrasound with Introduction by Esther Thaler," Video, 1983, https://www.youtube.com/watch?v=pkHrE2hUygU.

[127] David Rosenberg, "How to Remove Fear from Birth Culture" (TEDx, May 5, 2016), https://tedxinnovations.ted.com/2016/05/05/how-to-remove-fear-from-birth-culture/.

[128] TMR, "How I Gave My Son Autism," August 29, 2014, http://thinkingmomsrevolution.com/how-i-gave-my-son-autism/.

[129] "Spotting, Bleeding, Passing Clots after Transvaginal Ultrasound - February 2016 Babies," What To Expect, accessed March 6, 2016, http://www.whattoexpect.com/forums/february-2016-babies/topic/spotting-bleeding-passing-clots-after-transvaginal-ultrasound.html.

conducted when DUS intensity was generally low compared to present-day.

Clinicians see bleeding as insignificant, as Torrey states:

> *Mid-trimester bleeding was especially prevalent. The bleeding was usually minor and was not considered to be clinically significant at the time of occurrence.* [130]

Gao (2010), a controlled laboratory study, found maternal bleeding following transvaginal DUS. Gao also found DUS damage to the chorionic villi.[131]

As usual, Modern Medicine puts its hand right back in the cookie jar. Transvaginal ultrasound is the method of evaluation abnormal uterine bleeding, and the treatment advised is surgery or birth control pills.[132]

The negative health implications are vast for the individual and society. DUS appears to have set the human species on a tragic path due to its subtle and not-so-subtle biological effects. Critics argue that the exponential rise in autism incidence is largely the

---

[130] E. F. Torrey, S. P. Hersh, and K. D. McCabe, "Early Childhood Psychosis and Bleeding during Pregnancy. A Prospective Study of Gravid Women and Their Offspring," *Journal of Autism and Developmental Disorders* 5, no. 4 (January 1, 1976): 287–97.

[131] Su Fang Gao and Zuo Li, "Apoptosis And Restoration Of Human Villi During First Trimester Pregnancy After Exposure To Transvaginal Ultrasound" (Clinical Hospital of Tianjin Medical University, 2010), http://www.globethesis.com.

[132] Andrew M. Kaunitz, MD, "Abnormal Uterine Bleeding," August 19, 2015, http://www.uptodate.com/contents/abnormal-uterine-bleeding-beyond-the-basics.

result of fetal exposure to ultrasound.[133,134] If they are correct, then it may take many generations to recover from this misguided application of medical technology. DUS damages DNA.

While this may seem alarming, it bears a similarity to the aforementioned WHO document, "Criteria 22". Many scientists worldwide signed the document, including Wesley Nyborg, PhD, of the U.S. Food and Drug Administration (FDA), Melvin Stratmeyer, PhD, of the FDA, and William O'Brien, Jr., PhD, of the Bioacoustics Research Laboratory, University of Illinois:

> *...more than 35 published animal studies suggest that in utero ultrasound exposure can affect prenatal growth...* A number of biological effects have been observed *following ultrasound exposure in various experimental systems. These include reduction in immune response, change in sister chromatid exchange frequencies, cell death, change in cell membrane functions, degradation of macromolecules, free radical formation, and reduced cell reproductive potential... The data on clinical efficacy and safety* ***do not allow a recommendation for routine screening...***

The WHO Criteria was published 34 years ago. Its concerns have never been refuted. These concerns are supported by most modern science, though to date, that science has not been acknowledged by the dominant politic. What was described by WHO as an unacceptable risk three decades ago is now a much greater risk because the FDA has since raised its allowed machine intensities by a factor of 8x to 15x.

---

[133] Caroline Rodgers, "Questions about Prenatal Ultrasound and the Alarming Increase in Autism," Midwifery Today, no. 80 (Winter 2006), http://www.midwiferytoday.com/articles/ultrasoundrodgers.asp.

[134] Jack Rabin, MD, *Ultrasound and Autism: What Every Pregnant Woman Should Know*, 1st edition (Medical Discourse, 2015).

NEWNHAM (1993)

Newnham (1993) is a human exposure study with two followup studies on later child development. The studies concern children exposed *in utero* during the years 1989-1991. A total of 2,834 maternal-fetal pairs were exposed to DUS from early generation machines at low ultrasound intensity. Many sessions were at less than 5mW/cm2 SPTA, none more than 25mW/cm2 SPTA.[135] Disease was found.

> *Our findings suggested that [five or more ultrasound sessions] increase the proportion of growth-restricted fetuses by about one third. ...it would seem prudent to limit ultrasound examinations of the fetus...*[136]

These observations of growth restriction are important in that they were found despite the dismissal of dismiss data with statistical significance filters.

The study compared children from two groups of women exposed to DUS, a "regular" exposure group, and an "intensive" exposure group. The intensive group had more DUS sessions and higher exposure per session. The study results would have been much stronger had the study used a no exposure group. Omitting a no exposure group dilutes any observations of DUS hazards.

---

[135] SPTA, acronym for Spatial Peak Temporal Average. This is the standard intensity parameter for transducer output. There are many possible parameters. SPTA is defined as the maximum temporal average intensity for radiation. After 1991, SPTA was replaced in the machine display with two risk parameters, MI (Mechanical Index) and TI (Thermal Index). SPTA is generally considered better for discussion related to clinical exposure, and is used throughout this article.

[136] Newnham et al., "Effects of Frequent Ultrasound during Pregnancy."

Growth restriction makes sense as growth restriction had been found in earlier animal and cell studies.[137] Growth restriction is a big problem in itself and its presence implies a syndrome of possible malformations, neurological impairment, etc.[138]

Eight years later, Newnham followed up on the same population and published a study claiming that by year one, the size of smaller children had caught up to the norm, employing statistical significance arguments.

20 years later, Newnham followed up on the same population, studying intraocular development. It played down "differences" with statistical significance arguments:

> *There was no statistically significant difference between the two groups with regard to ocular biometric or visual outcomes...*[139]

However, most statisticians agree it is bad practice to omit data and discussion because of "statistical significance".

Schmidt & Hunter (2002), on statistical significance:

---

[137] W. D. O'Brien, Jr. and M. E. Stratmeyer, "Ultrasonically Induced Weight Reduction In Mice [1975]," *Congen Anomal* 15, no. 260 (1975).

[138] This finding of growth restriction does not exclude the possibility that DUS could also cause the opposite, i.e., macrosomia.

[139] H. Forward et al., "Multiple Prenatal Ultrasound Scans and Ocular Development: 20-Year Follow-up of a Randomized Controlled Trial," *Ultrasound in Obstetrics & Gynecology: The Official Journal of the International Society of Ultrasound in Obstetrics and Gynecology* 44, no. 2 (August 2014): 166–70, doi:10.1002/uog.13399.

> *Significance testing almost invariably retards the search for knowledge by producing false conclusions about research literature... a disastrous method for testing hypotheses.*

Newnham could not dismiss everything. It found a significant persistent disease:

> *...except for slightly higher intraocular pressure...*

That persisting ocular disease indicates that there are likely other unstudied diseases of unknown types, as the ocular disease is part of a larger DUS damage syndrome.

The defects observed by Newnham resulted after exposure to older machines, i.e., the defects resulted from low intensity DUS, ranging from less than 5mW/cm2 to 25mW/cm2. Newer machines, manufactured after 1991, range up to the 720mW/cm2 limit and sometimes higher.

STALBERG (2008)

This Swedish study reviews four population studies.[140] It is categorized here as an early work (before FDA/1991) despite being published in 2008 because it reviews the records of large populations of children who had been exposed to prenatal DUS during the 1970s and 1980s, the era of low intensity machines. It admits a dilution of its results due to its economy of design.

Stalberg finds some increased risk for boys (not girls) in the following categories: Schizophrenia, lower intellectual ability, lower

---

[140] K. Stalberg et al., "Prenatal Ultrasound Exposure and School Achievement in Teenagers; Follow-up of a Randomized Controlled Trial," *Ultrasound in Obstetrics and Gynecology* 32, no. 3 (2008): 306–306, doi:10.1002/uog.5602.

performance in school, lower performance in physical education, and a tendency towards left-handedness.

Stalberg concludes that the increased risks did not reach statistical significance, though with important exceptions, such as:

> *Boys exposed to ultrasound at any time during gestation had lower mean grades in physical education and a tendency towards lower school grades in general.*

Stalberg suggests that DUS may contribute to a general stress-induced vulnerability to disease:

> *Ultrasound and other prenatal and environmental events may be the elements that 'turn on' susceptibility genes in predisposed individuals.*

Thanks to Stalberg for their description of DUS-initiated fetal vulnerability, however, I will argue that it is not "turned-on" genes, but simple DUS damage that "predisposes" individuals to disease.

Stalberg provides a grim warning:

> *...these studies assessed ultrasound exposure in the 1970 and 1980s, with average intensity output levels for ultrasound machines of around 20 mW/cm2. This is very low compared to the maximum limit of 720 mW/cm2 set by the U.S. FDA... [clinical] outputs are probably ten times higher today... Further, the intensities for ultrasound machines are based on the manufacturer's data and high discrepancies have been found...*

Early Animal and Cell Studies

Siegel (1979) observed increased cell detachment at low exposure.[141] Cells normally attach to substrates and to each other. Their finding relates to embryo implantation problems and fetal growth restriction. Siegel was mentioned in WHO "Criteria 22" as a reason to deny routine DUS.

Cachon (1981) observed damage to cell microtubules with only 10 seconds exposure[142] of pulsed ultrasound at a low intensity of 8mW/cm2.[143] The study was cited in WHO "Criteria 22" as a reason to deny routine DUS.

Ellisman (1987) observed myelination disruption at the extremely low intensity of 0.135mW/cm2. This is a rat pup study emulating the human fetal scenario. No serious discussion followed this devastating study of DUS. Though initially given a high quality rating by the NIH, it was later denied funding for continuation.

Beverley Beech, of AIMS-UK, characterizes the importance of animal studies:

> *Over the years there have been numerous studies on rats, mice and monkeys which have found reduced fetal weight in babies... in the monkey studies, the ultrasound babies sat or lay around the bottom of the cage, whereas the little control monkeys were climbing up the bars and were up to the usual monkey tricks... What happens when the monkeys grow up?... as Jean Robinson has pointed out,*

---

[141] E. Siegel et al., "Cellular Attachment as a Sensitive Indicator of the Effects of Diagnostic Ultrasound on Cultured Human Cells," no. 133 (1979): 175–79.

[142] J. Cachon, M. Cachon, and J.N. Bruneston, "An Ultrastructural Study of the Effects of Very High Frequency Ultrasounds on a Microtubular System (Axopods of a Heliozoan).," *Biol. Cell* 40, no. 69 (1981).

[143] Estimated SPTA from 2.5mW/cm2 SATA

monkeys do not learn to read, write, multiply, sing opera, or play the violin.[144]

FDA/1991: Allowed Intensities Rise

This historical event marks the huge increase in DUS intensities and various epidemics of childhood disease.

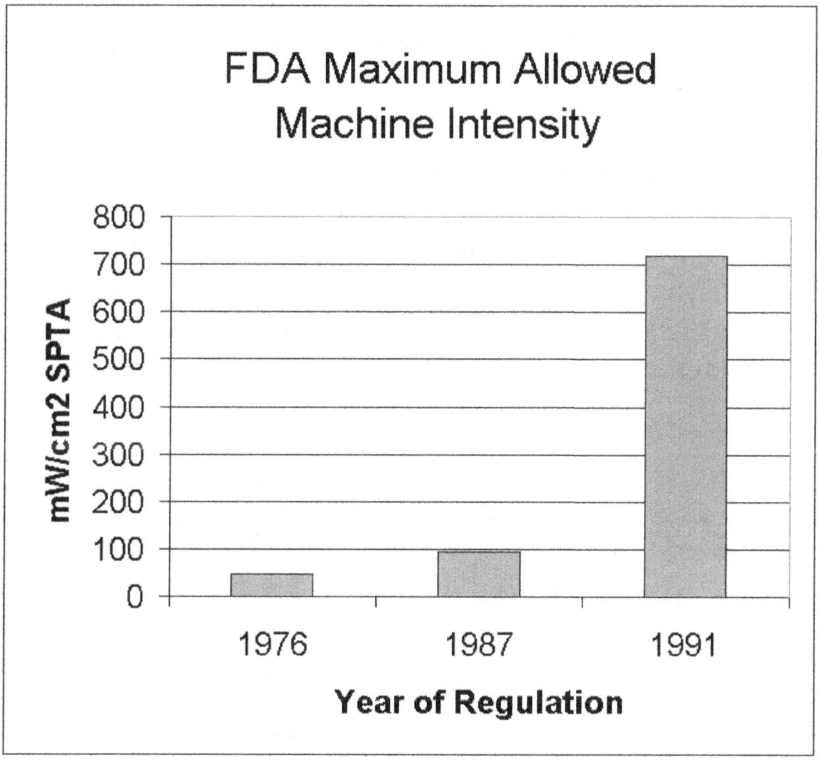

[144] Beverley Lawrence Beech, "Ultrasound - the Mythology of a Safe and Painless Technology," *A Paper Presented to the Royal Society of Medicine. Acknowledgement to Jean Robinson*, October 3, 1995, http://www.aims.org.uk/OccasionalPapers/ultrasoundTheMyth.pdf.

During 1991, FDA negotiations among "interested parties" resulted in an 8x-15x increase in allowable DUS machine intensities and with safety responsibility placed entirely on the operator.[145]

Since 1976, negotiations have always had a proposition on the table for unlimited machine intensities. Ostensibly, this is to facilitate industrial progress. DLMiller (2008):

> *[T]o liberalize the upper limit categories in some way to avoid inhibiting the development of diagnostic ultrasound...*[146]

FDA provides guidelines and special limits regarding intensity and exposure duration. However, these are weak, as the 720mW/cm2 limit applies to nearly all prenatal applications, even for the very sensitive eye of the fetus. This represents an absurdly dangerous paradox: The FDA intensity limit for the adult eye is 50mW/cm2, yet the intensity limit for the fetal eye is 720mW/cm2. DLMiller:

> *The new [DUS] limits were essentially made uniform across [application] categories,* ***except for [adult] opthalmological*** *examinations, for which consideration of possible heating indicated exceptional risk to the [adult] eye lens. The* ***obstetrical*** *ultrasound limit... was elevated to the highest 720 mW/cm2... the actual increases have not been as dramatic as these numbers indicate...*

My brackets and emphasis should not be necessary, i.e., DLMiller, if not under censure, presumably would have clearly described

---

145 Susan Katz Miller, "Summary: Exposure Criteria for Medical Diagnostic Ultrasound: II. Criteria Based on All Known Mechanisms" (National Council on Radiation Protection and Measurements, 2003)

146 Douglas L Miller, "Safety Assurance in Obstetrical Ultrasound," *Seminars in Ultrasound, CT, and MR* 29, no. 2 (2008): 156–64, doi:10.1053/j.sult.2007.12.003.

this paradox, but he conceals it from any naive readership. His language is self-neutering in that he minimally complies with the ethics of describing the dangerous contradiction.

Inappropriate Science

As intensities and disease incidence increased, did the NIH step up, appropriately funding studies?

No. The opposite. Only a few studies were conducted after 1991. In general, these studies found ultrasound hazardous but were denied funding for continuance, played down, and ignored.

From 1950 to the mid-1980s, there were over 700 studies reporting ultrasound-induced bioeffects, yet without resolution of human risk.[147]

Anderson and Barrett (1979):

> *The medical application of low-energy ultrasound as a diagnostic aid has developed in the* ***absence of appropriate*** *studies of its hazards.*

Ellisman (1987):

> *Several reviews of the literature... reveal that* ***most studies were inadequately designed*** *or inconclusive for the human medical situation; information on exposure conditions was frequently incomplete, markedly different from diagnostic ultrasound or in some instances sample size and follow-up were less than optimal.*

---

[147] Morton W. Miller and Victor Ciaravino, "Letters: Diagnostic Ultrasound, Miller, Caravino," *Science* 228, no. 4700 (May 10, 1985): 650, doi:10.1126/science.3857706.

No Science

Worse than inappropriate science is no science.

Abramowicz (2013):

> *for fetal imaging, the ISPTA was allowed to increase by a factor of almost 16 from 1976 and almost 8 from 1986 to 1992, yet...* ***all epidemiological information*** *available regarding fetal effects* ***predates 1992.***[148]

DLMiller (2012):

> *[As of 1992] the allowable output for obstetrical ultrasound was increased [8x-15x]... There has been little or* ***no subsequent research...*** *to systematically assess potential risks to the fetus...*[149]

DLMiller is authoritative, funded by the NIH. With his humble admission of "little or no research", he confirms the dismal state of ultrasound science. With his silence, however, he denies the dominant existence of science that indicts DUS. Most scientists do the same. They are quoted in DUS Book 1.

---

[148] Jacques S. Abramowicz, MD, "Bioeffects of Obstetric Ultrasound for the Clinician: How to Keep It Safe," *Institute For Advanced Medical Education*, February 2013.

[149] Douglas L. Miller et al., "Overview of Therapeutic Ultrasound Applications and Safety Considerations," *Journal of Ultrasound in Medicine* 31, no. 4 (April 1, 2012): 623–34.

Science vs Policy

See the following table, "Science vs Policy". Its exposure ratios provide a stunning measure of the disjunct between science and public policy.

	Science			Policy	
	Siegel	Cachon	Ellisman	AIUM (1987)	FDA (1991)
Seconds	30	10	1,800	500	500
Est Intensity (SPTA)	3	8	0.135	100	720
Exposure=T x I	90	80	243	50,000	360,000
Exposure Ratios					
AIUM : Science	556	625	206	1.0	0.1
FDA1991 : Science	4,000	4,500	1,481	7.2	1.0
Intensity Ratios					
AIUM : Science	33	13	741	1.0	0.1
FDA1991 : Science	240	90	5,333	7.2	1.0

The table contains three studies (Siegel, Cachon, and Ellisman) and two official policy statements (AIUM, FDA). The studies specify low intensities where damage was observed. The policies stated in the table specify intensities of official safety thresholds.

See "Exposure Ratios" in the table. With these ratios, I compare Science versus Policy. Ratios were calculated by dividing Policy Exposures by Science Exposures. Example: "50,000" divided by "90" equals "556".

As can be seen, the ratios are huge, i.e., the difference between Science and Policy is huge.

These three studies were selected for their low exposures. They have never been properly reviewed before being ignored. Example of impropriety: Del Cerro (1994) claims to have overturned Ellisman, but did not use Ellisman's expert methods. It claims to have duplicated Ellisman, but it did not.[150] Ellisman is a renowned neuroscientist. The lead author of Del Cerro (1994) is Morton W. Miller, a botanist, accused of incompetence and conflict of interest with the radiation industries, per the EMF epidemiologist, Dr. Milham, personal communication.

And, there is Andrew Marino, PhD, his critique of Miller:

> *With reference to performing experiments, he [MWMiller] stated, "I follow the golden rule - he who has the gold makes the rules."*[151]

Marino's quote is only one of many. It appears that the courts allowed Miller such statements without punishment or reprimand. Marino, as an expert environmental witness, often testifying against Miller. As Marino submitted papers to the court, he would occasionally forgot to include the "t" in Morton Miller's first name.

In the mainstream, there is no critical discussion regarding Del Cerro or Ellisman. Del Cerro is cited only when playing down Ellisman.[152]

The usual mainstream defense is:

> *"It is unlikely that a fetus would be exposed to such long dwell times."*

---

[150] Manuel Del Cerro et al., "A Test of the Hypothesis That Diagnostic Ultrasound Disrupts Myelination in Neonatal Rats," *Ultrasound in Medicine & Biology* 20, no. 9 (1994): 981–86, doi:10.1016/0301-5629(94)90057-4.

[151] Andrew Marino, PhD, "Point 12: The Testimony of Applicants' Witness Sol Michaelson Regarding the Health Hazards of High Voltage Transmission Lines Is Without Merit," March 6, 1976, http://andrewamarino.com/Testimonies/testimonymarino_4d.html.

[152] Personal communication with scientists, and my research of literature.

However, Cachon's dwell time is only 10 seconds. Siegel only 30 seconds. Ellisman, longer at 30 minutes (1,800 seconds), however, when Ellisman's extremely low intensity is extrapolated to the very high clinical intensities of present-day, dysfunction of myelination could be indicated within a few seconds exposure.

In 2013, the disjunct between public perception and scientific reality was described by Jacques Abramowicz, MD, a highly respected authority, professor, consultant to ultrasound machine manufacturers, and prestigious member of the American Institute of Ultrasound in Medicine (AIUM).[153]

> *If asked, the vast majority of end users (and patients) will respond that ultrasound is not X-rays and is completely safe. In reality, there is* ***a marked lack of knowledge*** *on effects of ultrasound in tissues being examined (bioeffects) among the majority of these end-users.* [154]

Profit adores "a marked lack of knowledge".

CONFIRMATION

DUS is not just a nightmare.

Mainstream experts generally agree that ultrasound has the potential to produce harmful biological effects in the fetus. For example, the WHO Criteria 22 describes risks as determined by animal and cell studies. Because these risks have not been confirmed

---

[153] AIUM, "American Institute of Ultrasound in Medicine", a multidisciplinary medical association of more than 9,000 physicians, sonographers, scientists, students, and other health care providers. Established in 1952, AIUM interfaces with industry, is a member of WFUMB, "The World Federation for Ultrasound in Medicine", a WHO organization.

[154] Jacques S. Abramowicz, MD, "Bioeffects of Obstetric Ultrasound for the Clinician: How to Keep It Safe."

by human studies, the practice of DUS continues, as the FDA, in 2013, definitively declared a contradiction:

> *Although **laboratory studies have shown** that diagnostic levels of ultrasound **can produce physical effects** in tissue, there is **no evidence from human studies of a causal relationship** between diagnostic ultrasound exposure during pregnancy and adverse biological effects to the fetus.*[155]

Political paradoxes

Funding for animal and cell laboratory studies has virtually disappeared from the Euro-American realm since the allowed machine levels were raised 8x in 1991.

I found four such studies, and they all indicate ultrasound to be considerable risk: Stanton (2001)[156], Ang (2006)[157], Krasovitski (2011)[158], Hočevar (2012), and most recently, Webb (2016).

---

[155] Sarah L. Cibull, BS, Gerald R. Harris, PhD, and Diane M. Nell, PhD, "Trends in Diagnostic Ultrasound Acoustic Output From Data Reported to the US Food and Drug Administration for Device Indications That Include Fetal Applications," J Ultrasound Med 32 (2013): 1921–32.

[156] MT Stanton et al., "Diagnostic Ultrasound Induces Change within Numbers of Cryptal Mitotic and Apoptotic Cells in Small Intestine," Life Sciences 68, no. 13 (February 16, 2001): 1471–75, doi:10.1016/S0024-3205(01)00940-7.

[157] Eugenius S. B. C. Ang et al., "Prenatal Exposure to Ultrasound Waves Impacts Neuronal Migration in Mice," Proceedings of the National Academy of Sciences 103, no. 34 (August 22, 2006): 12903–10, doi:10.1073/pnas.0605294103.

[158] Krasovitski et al., "Intramembrane Cavitation as a Unifying Mechanism for Ultrasound-Induced Bioeffects."

Stanton (2001), a mouse study, found increased cell death in the intestine at medium intensity DUS.[159] Funding was declined for continuation purposed to find lower thresholds.[160]

Ang (2006) caused public concern when it reported dysfunction of neuron migration in the brains of mice fetuses, caused by low intensity DUS.

The lead author, Pasko Rakic is a prominent neuroscientist at Yale University. In articles and interviews, he played down his own study. In 2010, it was reported that Rakic received funding for continuation in the form of another study, a monkey study. The funding was reported to be $3,000,000.[161] The rumor is that the study was completed, bioeffects were found, yet the study was quietly not published.

From an anonymous source:

> *[...Rakic] had positive results many years ago. Do not know why Pasko has sat on them.... the monkey studies. He did not cancel the same, just sat on the results.*

And,

> *...through the grapevine is that he received a lot of money to establish an endowment from a company that is tied to ultrasound equipment.*

---

[159] Stanton et al., "Diagnostic Ultrasound Induces Change within Numbers of Cryptal Mitotic and Apoptotic Cells in Small Intestine."

[160] Personal communications with Marie Stanton.

[161] Jim Giles, "Ultrasound Scans Accused of Disrupting Brain Development," *Nature* 431, no. 7012 (October 28, 2004): 1026–1026, doi:10.1038/4311026a.

Dr. Story, PhD, of the IACC, stated similarly,

> *...there was an initial report from Pasko Rakic in mice that ultrasound caused abnormalities in neuromigration and could represent a potential risk factor for autism. He has now replicated those studies, has done similar studies in primates, and hasn't published the results.* [162]

Story Landis, PhD, is Director of the National Institute for Neurological Disorders & Stroke, and IACC Member.

There are rumors as to why Rakic did not publish his well-funded study.

Hočevar (2012) is a high-tech rat study designed to approximate the human fetal scenario for DUS exposure. It studies cellular gene expression following low intensity DUS exposure. It unexpectedly found bioeffects similar to X-ray exposure, i.e., the gene GADD45a was several hundred times differentially expressed. Given that ultrasound radiation is not categorized as ionizing radiation (like X-rays), this was previously thought to be impossible.

Hočevar (2012) inadvertently supports the earlier research of Doreen Liebeskind, MD, at Columbia University, as follows.

Liebeskind (1981) is a cell study designed to be relevant to both clinical DUS and X-ray exposure. Ultrasound damage was similar to X-ray damage as observed under an electron microscope. When the results were extrapolated to a typical clinical session,

---

[162] IACC, "Strategic Plan Question 3: What Caused This To Happen and Can This Be Prevented? Responses.," *U.S. Dept Of Health And Human Services*, 2010, http://iacc.hhs.gov/public-comment/2010/rfi_comments/q3/index.shtml.

they indicated an equivalent risk of 250 chest X-rays.[163] A chest X-ray in 1981 was much higher intensity, i.e., much more destructive than present-day.

Liebeskind is thus even more relevant to present-day clinical sessions. Damage was permanent, heritable through cell division, demonstrating like Cachon (1981) that DUS exposure could conceivably affect many human generations. This is discussed in the WHO Criteria 22 as a reason not to endorse routine DUS.

Krasovitski (2011)[164] presents a sensitive mathematical model for ultrasound damage. The model was developed from the results of many experiments including its own experiments. Cellular damage was found at intensities 38x less than the FDA guideline of 1.9 MI (Mechanical Index).

Looking for the industrial defense to Krasovitski, I found that immediately after Krasovitski was published, the NIH funded a paper by Charles Church, PhD. He attempts to defend the FDA position with a refutation of Krasovitski.[165]

The professor overseeing Krasovitski is Eitan Kimmel, PhD, professor of biomedical engineering at the prestigious Technion Institute in Haifa, Israel.

---

[163] Doreen Liebeskind, MD et al., "Morphological Changes in the Surface Characteristics of Cultured Cells After Exposure to Diagnostic Ultrasound," Radiology 138 (February 1981): 419-23.

[164] Krasovitski et al., "Intramembrane Cavitation as a Unifying Mechanism for Ultrasound-Induced Bioeffects."

[165] Charles C. Church, "Theoretical Cavitation Thresholds in Vivo and Their Relationship to the Mechanical Index," The Journal of the Acoustical Society of America 131, no. 4 (April 1, 2012): 3385–3385, doi:10.1121/1.4708768.

Church never contacted EKimmel to clear up any possible misunderstandings. Church's paper consists largely of copy-pasted material with some old-school argument interspersed, and it ignores the import of EKimmel's supporting studies. Church cites 6 references. EKimmel cites 39 references. An updated version of EKimmel's study cites 45 references with several new experiments that provide additional support.[166] Yet, Church claims that EKimmel's models are unsupported by experiments.

Hazards Confirmed

In early 2013, I began my research for undeniable documentation. My motivation was due to an inability to convince people of DUS hazards with the existing critical material.

This frustration is widespread among critics. Emma Ashworth of AIMS-UK[167] relates a story of a midwife who informed all of her clients about the hazards of DUS. All except one still elected DUS.

I soon found, as described by the FDA and DLMiller, that only human studies are allowed as definitive evidence, and at the same time they are discouraged.

I then used a working theory: Somewhere there must be a study that employed a type of chromatography called "electrophoresis" to reveal ultrasound damage. This sensitive analytic technology uses a flow of mild electric current to enhance the separation of biochemical compounds during chromatography. Compounds visually separate. Electrophoresis is used, for example, to analyze

---

[166] Chen Geffen and Eitan Kimmel, "The Effect of Low Intensity Ultrasound on Adhesion Molecules, Actin Monomers and Membrane Permeability in Endothelial Cells," *Micro-Acoustics in Marine and Medical Research*, 2011.

[167] AIMS-UK stands for "Advancement for Improvements in Maternity Services", based in the United Kingdom. Much information about DUS can be found at www.aims.org.uk

DNA samples gathered from crime sites because DNA is unique to each person.

I wrote to ultrasound scientists, asking if they knew of an electrophoresis study, and I received no answer. I assumed there was no such study.

I persisted and eventually found JZhang (2002).[168] Not only was this an electrophoresis study, but it was a human study. Bonanza!

Through JZhang's references, and the references of his references, I was able to assemble a large number of arcane studies from the emerging online Chinese databases. I strove to gain a greater understanding of ultrasound science in order to competently evaluate and defend this finding from industry and plagiaristic corruption. I assembled the material as a book containing the new bibliography with extracts, commentary, illustrations, graphs and tables. I rewrote it as a more formal version, keeping only the essentials without speculation, shock and angst, to maintain stoic scientific tone. This was DUS Book 1.

Unknown to Western scientists and the public, the hazards of ultrasound to the human fetus have been confirmed in China since the late 1980s. This involved approximately 50 human studies, over 100 scientists, and 2,700 pregnant women (maternal-fetal pairs). Before abortion, they were exposed to carefully controlled DUS exposure levels, relevant to the clinical scenario. The studies were conducted over a period of 23 years, with the last, found so far, published in year 2011. These studies analyze abortive matter via electron-microscopy and biochemical assays.

---

[168] JiaYin Zhang et al., "Long Dwell-Time Exposure of Human Chorionic Villi to Transvaginal Ultrasound in the First Trimester of Pregnancy Induces Activation of Caspase-3 and Cytochrome C Release," *Biology of Reproduction* 67, no. 2 (August 1, 2002): 580–83, doi:10.1095/biolreprod67.2.580.

DUS Book 1 is an unprecedented East-West bridge, bringing essential arcana, the unknown Chinese Human Studies (CHS).

The CHS now allow us to say the previously unthinkable:

Human in utero dose/response studies are the most prevalent form of modern ultrasound science.

In this context, with the CHS and other appropriately designed studies, it would seem impossible that the practice of DUS could continue without major adjustments to protocols and machine settings.

The CHS began in 1988 with the presentation of a study of DUS bioeffects on human embryos. This occurred at a convention in Washington D.C. sponsored by the World Federation for Ultrasound in Medicine and Biology (WFUMB). With reference to the human studies, several Chinese scientists were presented an award during a special ceremony, Xin-Fang Wang, Yong-Chang Chou, Wang-Xue Guo, Zhi-Zhang Xu and Ruo Feng.[169]

[169] Xin-Fang Wang, "History of the Development of Ultrasound in China" http://www.ob-ultrasound.net/historychina.html.

The CHS continued with the encouragement of, arguably, the most influential ultrasound scientist in the United States at the time, Floyd Dunn, PhD.[170] In 1989, Dunn wrote a key letter to the most influential ultrasound scientist in China, Professor Ruo Feng, PhD, of Nanjing University. Feng was editor of the *Chinese Journal*

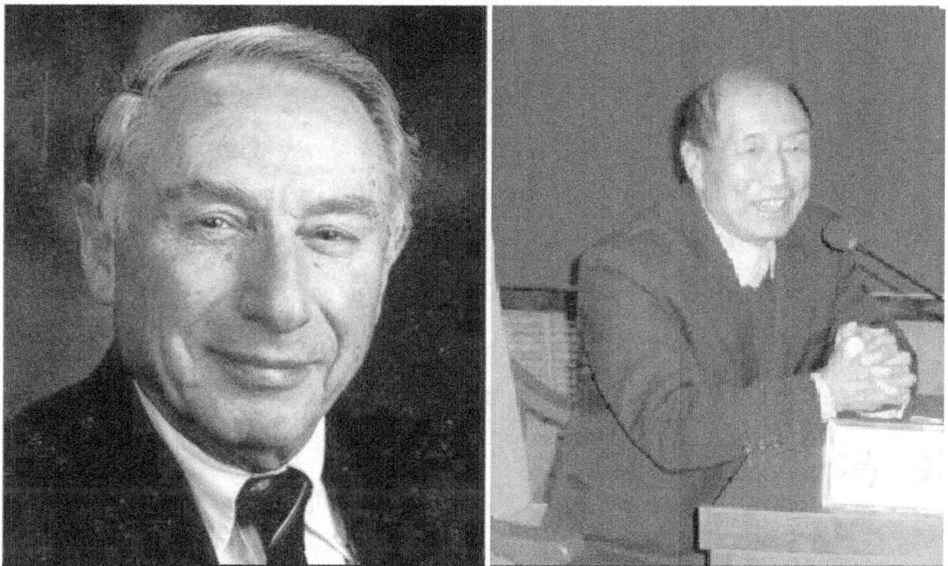

Floyd Dunn, PhD | Ruo Feng, PhD

of Ultrasound in Medicine, a member of editorial boards for journals internationally, and well known at ultrasound conventions throughout the world.[171] See photos.

---

[170] William D. O'Brien, Edwin L. Carstensen, and Wesley L. Nyborg, "Gold Medal Award 1998: Floyd Dunn," accessed December 22, 2013, http://acousticalsociety.org/about/awards/gold/12_10_10_dunn.

[171] Jim West, "Harvoa | Prof. Ruo Feng, Biography," Internet html, accessed March 11, 2016, http://harvoa.org/chs/rf.

In 1990, Feng published an overview of the hazards of DUS where he stresses the importance of the ongoing CHS. With an understanding of the political importance of Dunn's letter, Feng documented the letter in Chinese and English language.[172] See letter extract, with my highlight.

根本不可能进行的。如果在你们国家可以进行，那么依我之见，它对于国际诊断超声将是重大贡献。

(……This topic would be extremely difficult, possibly even impossible, to carry out in this country because of a prevailing view regarding abortion. If this could be carried out in your country, in my view, it would be a major contribution to international diagnostic ultrasound.)》

五、如周文与苗文所说，巩文在研究工作中使用了明显大于临床上常用的超声诊断剂量。因而由

With Dunn's encouragement, the Chinese continued the human studies project over the next two and a half decades. These studies cite and support the observations of several earlier studies in the Western realm.

Despite their scientific success, the CHS were not acknowledged. Dunn stayed silent. He is deceased as of January 24, 2015. Ruo Feng is retired and not in good health.

---

[172] Ruo Feng, "Ultrasonic Diagnostic Dose Intrauterine Fetal Embryos Security," *Chinese Journal of Ultrasound* 6, no. 3 (1990): 210–11.

JZhang (2002)

JZhang (2002) is the amazing electrophoresis study, a human *in utero* exposure study. The study is unknown and never discussed, like nearly all of the CHS, despite being published in pristine English and in modern scientific format.[173] The study finds DNA fragmentation in the chorionic villi caused by low intensity DUS at only 10 minutes exposure.

JZhang's observations are so strong that damage could be assumed probable at less than 10 minutes. Given that clinical sessions are conducted at much higher intensities, a simple extrapolation to the clinical scenario could indicate damage within seconds, not minutes. The chorionic villi comprise the essential nutrient-waste exchange apparatus between mother and fetus.

See the image, rendered from JZhang that represents DNA fragmentation caused by DUS exposure at four different time durations.

---

[173] JiaYin Zhang et al., "Long Dwell-Time Exposure of Human Chorionic Villi to Transvaginal Ultrasound in the First Trimester of Pregnancy Induces Activation of Caspase-3 and Cytochrome C Release."

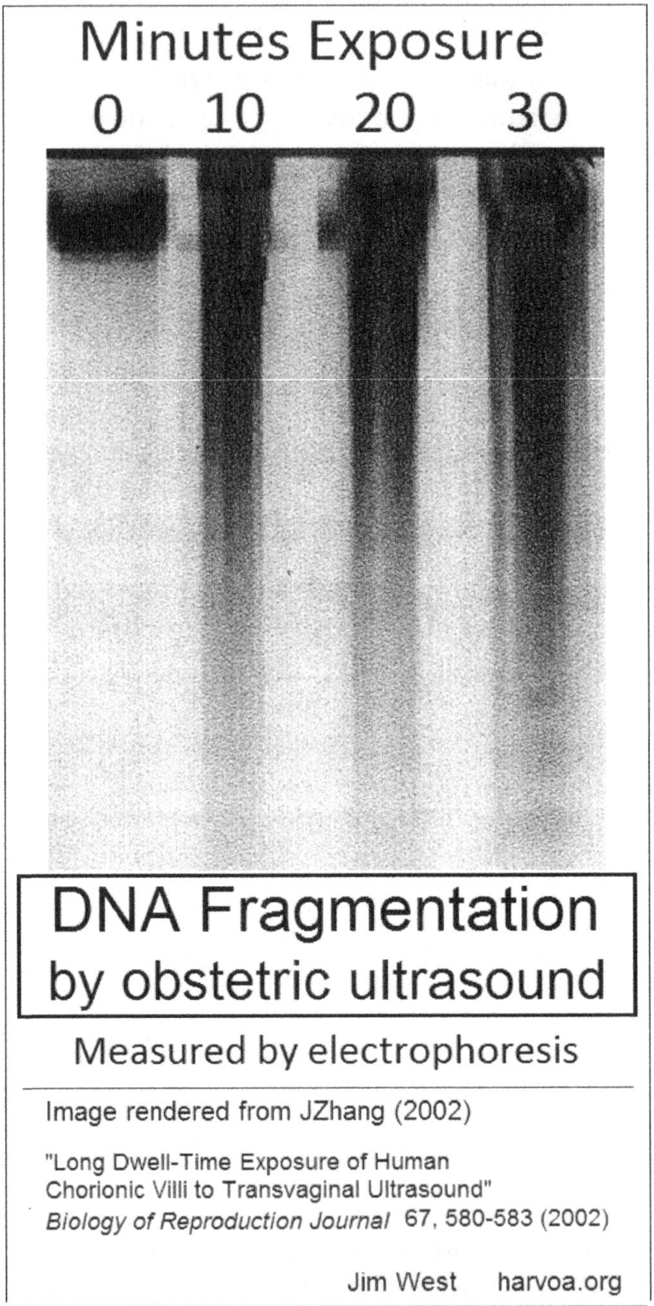
Minutes Exposure
0 10 20 30
DNA Fragmentation
by obstetric ultrasound
Measured by electrophoresis
Image rendered from JZhang (2002)
"Long Dwell-Time Exposure of Human
Chorionic Villi to Transvaginal Ultrasound"
Biology of Reproduction Journal 67, 580-583 (2002)
Jim West harvoa.org

At the end of 2014, I brought JZhang (2002) to the attention of the prominent ultrasound scientist, William O'Brien, Jr., PhD. With input from his colleague, Jacques Abramowicz, MD, O'Brien immediately wrote an article for publication, describing JZhang as an important study requiring serious attention. A review of JZhang was also expected from the AIUM Bioeffects Committee.

O'Brien's publication date and a Committee review have only been recently announced, with publication possibly imminent. I will monitor this if and when possible. Despite O'Brien's strong reputation, progress has been slow. Since 2002, JZhang's publication date, it has now been 14 years for this possibility of mainstream recognition.

JZhang is supported by many similar CHS, as described in DUS Book 1. DNA fragmentation would also relate to the fetus, as the fetus is intimate to the chorionic villi.

JZhang has huge implications for the present epidemic of chorioamnionitis, an inflammation of the chorion and amnion membranes in pregnant women (fetal and maternal junction membranes). Causation for this disease has been declared infection despite a frequent failure to associate germs with this disease.

JZhang has huge implications for many childhood diseases, for example, the present-day emergence of childhood cancers and leukemia. DNA fragmentation happens to be the foremost theory for cancer causation.[174] The epidemic of neonatal jaundice should be considered because the CHS confirm the older Euro-American

---

[174] Elzbieta Pawlowska and Janusz Blasiak, "DNA Repair—A Double-Edged Sword in the Genomic Stability of Cancer Cells—The Case of Chronic Myeloid Leukemia," International Journal of Molecular Sciences 16, no. 11 (November 18, 2015): 27535–49, doi:10.3390/ijms161126049.

studies that found dysfunction of immune systems caused by DUS. Those studies were discussed in the WHO Criteria 22.

The CHS are human studies of *in utero* fetal exposure to diagnostic ultrasound. These generally exceed the legacy of Western science in terms of technical sophistication, era relevancy, volume of work, and number of subjects. They bring empirical human evidence for ultrasound hazards.

The CHS are simple. Pregnant women, volunteering for abortion, were carefully selected then exposed to controlled ultrasound sessions, using standard clinical devices at various intensity settings and exposure durations. Abortive matter was then examined via state-of-the-art technology (electron microscopy, flow cytometry, and various biochemical analyses (immuno- and histo-). The observations were compared against a control group.

The CHS measure DUS damage to the fetal brain, kidney, cornea, chorionic villi, and immune system. They determined that low exposure is able to damage the human fetus, ovum, and embryo.

Conclusion

What could be a more clear and undeniable damnation of DUS?

Why are clinicians instructed to expose the fetus to this controversial form of radiation during early gestation, during a period of rapid cellular division, of well-known vulnerability to ultrasound?

Why do clinicians expose the fetus to radiation knowing it is a hazard?

Why is DUS routinely advocated for determination of pregnancy, thereby ensuring higher risk?

These questions, posed long ago by the history of X-rays on pregnant women, remain unresolved.

Many professionals recognize DUS hazards, but they claim the greater hazard is birth without DUS. This brings an innate contradiction, as their views are often determined from assessments of data gathered from DUS examinations. Such assessments seem bizarre, given the evidence that DUS itself is teratogenic.[175] The mainstream inability to mention the obvious brings suspicion.

CATCH-22

The Euro-American realm generally declares,

- Only human studies can resolve the DUS controversy.
- Few human studies exist.
- For ethical reasons, human studies should not exist.[176]

Deconstructing this institutional gridlock...

Human studies are two types:

- Epidemiological reviews, i.e., population studies.
- *in utero* or *in vivo* exposure studies, such as the CHS, where abortive matter is evaluated in a laboratory following carefully controlled DUS exposure to the mother's ova, embryo, or fetus.

Epidemiological studies that exonerate DUS should be approached skeptically. They are complex and thus vulnerable to bias and exploitation. Tweaking is common in all types of science studies due to industrial imperatives. Epidemiologists have stated

---

[175] Teratogenic: Able to disturb the development of an embryo or fetus.

[176] This is my general overview as determined from my review of many statements by ultrasound scientists. A few of these are quoted in this article and many are quoted in my book. These are generalizations and there are exceptions such as Newnham (1993).

that tweaking studies down is common and acceptable practice in order to gain publication:

> *We are of course aware of the problems of biased re-porting of epidemiologic data in order to increase the chances of having the paper accepted...*[177]

There is already mainstream agreement that animal and cell studies demonstrate that ultrasound has the potential to damage the human fetus. Scientists claim they are waiting for confirmation from human studies, for example,

SHANKAR (2011)

> *The potential for ultrasound to cause adverse effects in experimental animals is well established, but whether similar effects also occur with humans in susceptible tissue (e.g., neural) requires further investigation...*
>
> *No human investigations conducted to date have documented major physiologic consequences of ultrasound exposed during imaging... The relative safety of ultrasound has been well established based on its use... over several decades...*
>
> *One could postulate that humans are resistant to ultrasound-related biologic effects...*[178]

---

[177] Jorn Olsen, Shah Ebrahim, and Chitr Sitthi-amorn, "Scientific Fraud and Epidemiology IEA," June 2013, http://ieaweb.org/2006/01/scientific-fraud-and-epidemiology/.

[178] Hariharan Shankar and Paul S. Pagel, "Potential Adverse Ultrasound-Related Biological Effects: A Critical Review," Anesthesiology 115, no. 5 (November 2011): 1109–24, doi:10.1097/ALN.0b013e31822fd1f1.

Shankar describes the present-day absurd mainstream consensus. DUS safety is "based on its use" with the medical industry in conflict of interest and science in unresolved contradiction. Humans in the clinical scenario are presumed "resistant" to bioeffects observed in cell and animal studies. Stasis is maintained with the Catch-22.

The ethical concern over human studies is false because abortion has long been legal, ethical and ubiquitous in the Western realm. Placental pathology is a well-established discipline. Appropriate science could have begun decades ago by merely including the toxicology of DUS into placental pathology.

There is a lot more to say. *A New Bibliography* presents a strong authoritative challenge to the industrial establishment. This should bring a serious reconsideration of the risk/benefit of ultrasound practice. The book,

- ***Introduces the Chinese Human Studies***, and reviews the prior status quo.
- ***Supports Western critics*** who have long argued that ultrasound contributes to child disease epidemics.
- **Revives Western cell and animal studies** that indicate ultrasound hazards.
- ***Enables toxicological arguments for childhood disease causation***, e.g., GI tract dysfunction, immune dysfunction, rashes, cancer, leukemia, and a wide variety of diseases related to wide-spectrum hormone and cell dysfunction.
- ***Describes how to minimize*** unavoidable DUS.
- ***Presents*** **an** ***Ultrasound Toxic Synergy Model***: This resolves contradictions within the anti-vax position.

Glossary

Autism Spectrum Disorder (ASD): A collection of disorders and syndromes, characterized by deficits in social interaction and limited, repetitive patterns of behavior.

Central Nervous System (CNS): The brain, spinal cord, and optic nerve.

The Chinese Human Studies (CHS): Studies of diagnostic ultrasound conducted circa 1988-2011.

Chorioamnionitis: An inflammation of the two adjacent fetal membranes that make up the amniotic sac. These are the chorion (maternal) and amnion (fetal) membranes, which together serve as the maternal-fetal nutrient-waste junction.

Comorbidity: The existence of multiple symptoms (or disorders) in the same organism, e.g., microcephaly, intrauterine growth restriction (IUGR), ocular defects, autism and ADHD.

Conflict of Interest: Where interests conflict with ethics.

Congenital: Present at birth, such as a birth defect or disorder, or a condition existing at birth.

Congenital Rubella Syndrome (CRS): A set of newborn disorders caused by a supposed rubella virus. These disorders potentially include microcephaly, vision, hearing, and neurological disorders, often correlating with ADHD and ASD.

Congenital microcephaly: A newborn condition where the infant's brain is abnormally small.

Congenital Zika Syndrome (CZS): A set of newborn disorders, potentially including microcephaly, vision, hearing, and neurological disorders (anticipated to include ADHD, ASD, etc.), caused by a supposed Zika virus.

Control group: A zero exposure group. A less exposed group. This group is compared to other more exposed groups in order to determine the dose/response effects of a suspected disease-causing agent.

Diagnostic ultrasound (DUS): An acoustic echo-imaging technology used for clinical diagnostics.

Epigenetic: Concerning the mutation of genes by the environment.

Electromagnetic fields (EMF): Fluctuating EMF is a health hazard, a form of radiation. Example of low frequency sources are alternating current from powerlines, electric motors, transformers, etc. In the high frequency range, there are radar systems, fluorescent lights, mobile phones, radio waves, X-rays, etc.

Epidemiological study: A population study of disease phenomena.

FDA: The Food and Drug Administration (U.S.)

Known: Generally accepted belief.

Germ theory: The belief that infectious predatory germs (viruses, bacteria, fungi, etc) are a major cause of disease.

Heritability: The extent to which genetic differences contribute to individual differences.

Iatrogenia: Medical causation of disease.

Incidence vs Prevalence: Incidence is the rate of disease occurrence. Prevalence is the fraction representing the diseased population.

Ionizing radiation: As defined by OSHA, "Any electromagnetic or particulate radiation capable of producing ion pairs by interaction with matter... [e.g., X-rays, gamma rays, etc.]" This excludes ultrasound, a form of acoustic radiation categorized as non-ionizing radiation.

Industry: (My redefinition) Polluting and exploiting industries. Beneficial industries (or corporations) are common, but not within my critical focus.

Known: Officially recognized as true.

Mainstream Media: Mainstream propaganda, e.g., news, internet content, films, plays, fiction and non-fiction, etc., funded by and beholden to industry for its health, often at odds with individual health.

Modern Medicine: A humorous term popularized by Dr. Robert S. Mendelsohn, former chair of the hospital licensing board for the State of Illinois. This term is synonymous with Mainstream Medicine.

Mutagen: An agent that causes a genetic mutation or changes the frequency of mutations.

Neonate: The first 28 days of a full-term infant's life.

Neonatology: A specialty of pediatrics; medical care of newborn infants, especially the ill or premature, usually hospital-based in the NICU. Combines with perinatology.

NIAID: National Institute of Allergy and Infectious Diseases.

NICU: Neonatal Intensive Care Unit.

OFC: Occipital Frontal Circumference, meaning Head Circumference (HC).

Original Sin Doctrine: (My redefinition) Doctrine that places the onus of guilt on the individual, thereby protecting and enabling hazardous industry. Examples of Original Sin: Bad genes, bad germs spread by sneezing, poverty, and supposed ignorance.

Pathogen: Any agent that causes disease. In practice, this term is usually biased to mean non-toxicological agents, e.g., germs or mutated genes.

Pediatrics: The field of medicine concerned with the health of children from birth to young adulthood. This is neonatal, though there is a prenatal loophole, as pediatrics includes prevention.

Perinatal: The period from 20 weeks before birth to 4 weeks after birth.

Phenylketonuria (PKU): An inherited newborn disorder of the metabolism that, when left untreated can lead to mental disorders, musty smell, seizures, heart defects, microcephaly and low birth weight. This disease was discovered in 1934.

Postnatal: The period following birth, up to six weeks.

Prenatal: Before birth, relating to pregnancy, antenatal.

P-value: The probability of an event occurring due to chance.

Roentgen rays: X-rays, a form of ionizing radiation.

Spectrum: A collection of symptoms, disorders, conditions, diseases, and/or syndromes.

Stillbirth: Death in the womb after 28 weeks gestation, or during birth. Death during the third trimester or birth. (WHO)

Teratogen: An agent that causes structural abnormality of the ova, embryo or fetus, other than a mutagen.

Therapeutic ultrasound: Ultrasound used as a treatment, e.g., to accelerate bone or muscle growth for repair. Usually the transducer output intensity is higher than diagnostic ultrasound (DUS).

Toxicological Avoidance (My term): The avoidance of toxicological topics by way of a myopic focus upon genes or germs. Toxicological Avoidance is Modern Medicine's primary role, the means by which it protects industry and avails exploitation.

Wikipedia: Known for clarity, *Wikipedia* is the most popular representative of mainstream belief. It is a measure of orthodoxy. Its rules demand the reinforcement of mainstream perception. Industrial interest monitors Wikipedia pages.

Author

Jim West attended Arizona State University, majoring in mechanical engineering and music composition/performance. He is autodidact in virology, toxicology, organic chemistry, and electronics.

Following three years in the U.S. military, Jim moved to New York City, where he became involved in computer consultancy, environmental research, politics, and the arts. He served as Chair of the Science Committee for the NoSpray Coalition, which litigated extensively against the Giuliani Administration with regard to the helicopter-driven pesticide spray programs that began circa 1999 re the West Nile epidemic. He is a member of Toastmasters and on the Advisory Board for *Discovery Salud*.

Jim's published work describes unprecedented discoveries of environmental causation for the great epidemics of polio, West Nile, SARS, Bird flu, etc. Several professional medical books have used his work with permission. In 2001, Nicholas Regush, producer and journalist for *ABC News*, wrote an in-depth article, "West Nile: Virus or Environment?", describing Jim's discovery of unpublicized MTBE petrochemical air pollution that had been severely increasing air pollution levels in the New York City region. The article was well received. There was talk of bringing Jim's work to ABC's evening shows such as *20/20* and *Nightline*, with ABC's "top brass" interested in Jim's work.

Copyright

ISBN 978-1-941719-08-4
Library of Congress Control Number: 2017944068

Contact
pub@harvoa.org
or
www.harvoa.org/contact

Made in the USA
Monee, IL
13 September 2026

62976617R00125